The Last Two Years

The Last Two Years

A Difficult Journey of Mind, Body and Soul As seen through the Prism of an Ovarian Cancer Survivor's Husband

Arthur Marsicano

iUniverse, Inc.
New York Lincoln Shanghai

The Last Two Years
A Difficult Journey of Mind, Body and Soul As seen through the
Prism of an Ovarian Cancer Survivor's Husband

Copyright © 2006 by Arthur Marsicano

iUniverse books may be ordered through booksellers or by
contacting:

iUniverse
2021 Pine Lake Road, Suite 100
Lincoln, NE 68512
www.iuniverse.com
1-800-Authors (1-800-288-4677)

The views expressed herein are the sole responsibility of the author
and do not necessarily reflect the views of iUniverse or its affiliates.

ISBN-13: 978-0-595-41318-8 (pbk)
ISBN-13: 978-0-595-67894-5 (cloth)
ISBN-13: 978-0-595-85671-8 (ebk)
ISBN-10: 0-595-41318-8 (pbk)
ISBN-10: 0-595-67894-7 (cloth)
ISBN-10: 0-595-85671-3 (ebk)

Printed in the United States of America

Dedicated to Lucas Fredericks
Born and died on Saint Patrick Day, March 17, 2000

Pop Pop will always love you

AUTHOR'S NOTES

Great care was taken to confirm all factual information presented in the book. However, there is one aspect of the book that is not entirely accurate. Individuals have a right to privacy; consequently, actual names were not always used. In some cases even the names of locations and organizations were altered.

This book does not contain medical advice! Nothing in this book should be considered a suggestion, recommendation, or endorsement of any medicine, medical procedure, physician, hospital, medical professional, or medical organization. The author assumes no responsibility for any medical action the reader engages in whether through self-care or under the care of a medical professional. Anyone suffering from cancer or any other illness should consult with a licensed healthcare professional for all medical advice and treatment.

TABLE OF CONTENTS

Part One

INTRODUCTION

The last two years have been very difficult for my family. During this time my father died after a long period during which his health slowly, but continually, declined. Simultaneously, my wife of forty years experienced a series of serious medical problems, including cancer. After my father's death, I felt a need to write a description of the journey my wife and I had taken over the last two years. But this was not a journey in any conventional sense. It was a difficult and painful journey of the mind, body, and soul that we took along the same path in the physical world while we traveled separately with understanding and compassion for each other, in the more complex and equally important worlds of the mind and soul.

I am writing this book because I recognize that many people and many families also face times of deep despair. The path my wife and I traveled is described in this book and should provide those who read it with comfort and some useful insights when they find themselves on their own difficult journey of the mind, body, and soul.

CHAPTER 1
God, Religion, and the Spiritual World

This book presents a true account of a two-year period in the life of a cancer survivor—my wife Jean Marsicano. I was with her during the entire period, sharing the emotions and the drama that was played out. While the book focuses on events in Jean's life, other family members, friends and dear souls Jean and I came into contact with were also facing life-altering experiences. It was not a typical two year period … not by any stretch of the imagination. So much happened that it was difficult—no impossible—to present all of the emotions and *"cross currents of events"* that took place.

Jean and I have had strong but different views about God, religion and the spiritual world from the time we were married to the present. Like most people, we *"took God for granted."* Faced with the certainty of my father's death and the possibility of Jean's, we focused as never before on *"God."* We hoped, we prayed, we cried, and we talked frequently about God, death and life after death. We also considered our lives. Did we accomplish anything of value? Did our lives have meaning?

I am not a religious person, *at least not in any traditional sense.* However, the search for God and things spiritual in nature are

extremely important to me; but organized religion is less important. I have enormous respect for all religions, not just the one I
belong to, but I do not feel obligated to accept the teachings or
beliefs of any of them. *I believe what I believe*! My views are complex and unique, and they created difficulty for me as I wrote this
book. I know there are inconsistencies and biases in my opinions
and beliefs regarding all things spiritual, and this will be obvious
to the reader. I simply can not separate my beliefs from my writing. Consequently, it would be difficult to appreciate this book
without some understanding of how my spiritual beliefs and
views evolved. Recognizing this, I wrote the following statement
and offer it for your consideration……. *"God Was There"* ….

God Was There

At the beginning of the long march of history, humanity searched for the meaning of its existence and found God, an eternal presence greater than all that was.

Four thousand years ago God was there when the most enduring of religions began in a region that came to be known as the Holy Lands.

God was there when the Romans crucified a holy man and when his followers spread his teachings and the record of his life and death.

God was there when Mohammed wrote the inspired words of the Koran and with those who spread Islam across Africa and the Middle East. And God was there as Islam threatened Christian Europe.

God was there when the Christian world discovered and seized the New World, and God was there when Christians destroyed the cultures of that world, and did it in the name of Christ.

God was there when a great man said, "This nation under God shall have a new birth of freedom" as part of an address that has inspired many as it echoes through the ages.

God was there in the heart and soul of Mahatma Gandhi when he organized a brilliant non-violent resistance against British occupation of his beloved India and when he said:

"I consider myself a Hindu, Christian, Muslim, Jew, Buddhist and Confucian."

God was there as the world built by Communist atheists collapsed when confronted by a courageous demand for justice relent-

lessly pursued by three men of God: a Pope who will one day be a saint, an American President who loved to smile, and a humble Polish union member. Earlier, God was there as the Pope and the President miraculously survived assassin bullets.

God was there when Islamic terrorists murdered 3,000 innocent people on American soil. Their God was a God of Hate that has never been able to defeat the God of Love.

God was there. God will always be there. Cultures that fail to accept this will decline, and individuals who ignore the possibility of God will be unable to appreciate the joys of life and endure the pain and sorrow we must all experience.

God and the Long March of History

Throughout history humanity's search for God played an essential role that continues to this day. Christian Europe was threatened and contained by Islam until the discovery of the New World allowed Europe and Christianity to expand and increase its power at the expense of Islam and the rest of the world. Christianity was the essential ingredient utilized by the nations of Europe to gain control of most of North and South America initially and later most of the rest of the world. For many years, it was correctly said, *"The Sun Never Sets on The British Empire."* Obviously the British were not the only Europeans to colonize and exploit the rest of humanity, but they did it more effectively than the rest of Europe. Domination of much of the world by the Christian nations of Europe began around 1600 AD and did not end for more than 300 years; indeed some vestiges of it exist even today.

The Long March of History can not be appreciated without an understanding of humanity's search for God. Similarly, this book can not be understood without an appreciation of how the central players in the book relate to God, religion or a *"presence in the universe greater than all of humanity."* This book deals with a period of despair faced by an entire family. During such times many people turn to *"God and religion,"* as was the case with my family. People view and utilize God and religion in very different ways to ease their pain. Surprisingly, even those who are atheists may be forced to confront spiritual issues because the people around them may insist they make accommodations with God, if only for the sake of family and friends.

God or a Greater Presence

I am troubled by many aspects of organized religion, and I know others are as well. Even the word "God" troubles me at times because it seems too certain, too focused, too human, and perhaps even too Christian! I prefer to think of God as "a Greater Presence" because for me that encompasses all possibilities and all religions. In addition, the phrase "a Greater Presence" preserves the required strength and respect while remaining consistent with my feelings and beliefs. If God exists, then surely it is the same God that all people worship, including those who do not feel the need to worship God in a building surrounded by others of the same beliefs. Many people see and even feel a Greater Presence in the world around them. I feel it when I look at my grandchildren; when I walk the beaches of South Carolina; when I watch a powerful storm; and when I see a mother holding her baby.

During times of great pain people turn to God but usually to a God they have allowed their religion to interpret for them, rather than the God that is within them. As they experience pain they ask why it is happening to them or to their loved ones. *"Why do bad things happen to good people?"* or *"How could God allow this to happen?"* Some will even express anger or hatred toward their religion or God. During the last two years my family experienced my father's declining health and his death, and we lived with the uncertainty of my wife's health. Through it all, each of us looked to God—*each of us in our own way.*

Pain and Uncertainty

In my professional life I was employed as an engineer and as a university professor. Consequently, my writing was highly structured and predictable to the point of boredom. In contrast, when I communicated orally, especially in front of a group of college students, I tried to stimulate thinking, entertain *(if possible)* and provide a basis for informed, intelligent debate. *(God, how I love a good debate!)* My oral presentations would not follow an orderly straight line approach because that would only result in boredom, and learning can not take place in the absence of interest.

Life, like my verbal communications, is rarely well organized, predictable, or orderly. This book is a message of hope embedded in a period of great pain and uncertainty. During times of great pain and anguish there can be, and should be, intervals of joy. Usually the joy will surface in some unexpected way, but it should be embraced and fully appreciated, even if the worst possible outcome is a certainty. Reviewing events of the last two years, I came face to face with issues that were deeply troubling to me. The nature of God, Jean's mortality, and my own mortality were unavoidable issues I considered. This took place at the core of my intellect and in another place: my soul. My writing will attempt to reflect all of this and the inner thoughts and fears that raced through my mind during this period.

I am conflicted about God and religion; I am not even sure that God exists. Nevertheless, I draw great strength from all things spiritual and from a hope there is a God associated with the Greater Presence I frequently feel around me. I am surprised I can draw strength from uncertainty, for I pride myself on being logical and analytical.

Offend No Person or Group

It is difficult to write or speak about God, religion, and life after death without offending individuals or even entire groups of people. I knew when I began writing this book that my words could offend many people, even friends and family members who know I mean no harm and know I respect all religions. Recognizing this danger, I will refrain from discussing the specifics of any religion.

I often describe and interpret the world metaphorically, for this compresses complex and even painful ideas into words that are more easily understood and in many cases less controversial. In addition, metaphors frequently have a universal meaning that can be readily understood by diverse groups. For example, I prefer the expression *"cross the river for the last time"* to other more direct, often painful, ways of describing death. In addition, *"crossing the river for the last time"* implies *"life after death,"* which is not the case for more direct expressions such as *"when I die"* or *"while in the final moments of life."* In this book I shall frequently rely on metaphors, for there are so many beautiful ones that deal with God, religion, and life after death. Furthermore, metaphors usually lack the specifics that could offend *"people of faith."*

In addition to my concern about offending *people of faith,* I have a concern about offending people identified in this book specifically by name or indirectly by other means. I assure all readers that there is absolutely no intention to embarrass or harm anyone. Indeed, I have nothing but good will toward every person mentioned in this book.

CHAPTER 2

My Prism and a Greater Presence

Each of us views life through our own prism, which is the result of our abilities, experiences and a unique "life spark" that has nothing to do with abilities or experiences. I am not certain that God exists, but I am certain that every man, woman, and child who ever existed or ever will exist, has a uniqueness that can not be explained. The above may seem a contradiction, especially since I believe it is likely our unique *life spark* was given to us by *a Greater Presence.* For me, any honest examination of God, religion, and life after death is filled with uncertainty and contradictions. I also see uncertainty and contradictions in many others when dealing with these issues, including the many people of faith I know and love.

Our individual prisms convert truth and reality into perceptions that vary widely across people and over time. An atheist sees what I see but is convinced science, if given sufficient time and resources, is capable of explaining everything. I look at my grandchildren and the power and grandeur of nature and know they are wrong. Science can never explain the love I feel for family and the stirrings within me when I am moved by nature. Science can describe and explain an increasing number of complex relationships that are in the world around us, but it cannot explain how or why the rules and equations that govern our world came into existence.

Every scientific discovery produces at least as many questions as answers. If you doubt this, ask a scientist when all of science will be known and the process of scientific discovery will come to an end. The answer is NEVER!

While writing these words I am sitting at my favorite spot on the South Carolina beach listening to the sounds of the ocean. The ocean is a great mystery to me—it seems to roar even when it is calm. It is 3 pm on March 16, 2006, and I see several dolphins. It is early in the year to see these beautiful creatures and I am thankful they are here, for their appearance serves to enhance the possibility of a Greater Presence. *My wife would very likely say their arrival is "a sign from God."* She often speaks with certainty about the nature of God. I respect her religious pronouncements although I do not accept them. How I envy her certainty about God and all things spiritual. However, my feelings about religion, God and what I to refer to as *a Greater Presence*, may help explain why I am writing this book.

(As indicated earlier, I prefer the phrase "a Greater Presence" to the word "God." However, in this book I shall generally use the word "God," if only to make the reader feel more comfortable and the book more readable.)

The prism through which I see and interpret the world around me is largely the result of my personal search for God and my interactions with family, especially four family members who will be identified shortly. I have never been able to find a satisfactory description of God in any religion. Perhaps that is why I have been uncomfortable with *"organized religion"* most of my life. Nevertheless, I enjoy attending services in any *"house of God"* and I hope to one day attend Jewish, Hindu and Muslim religious services; for if God exists, then God is present in every house of worship created by every religion.

Mahatma Gandhi was a towering figure of the 20th century influencing political and religious leaders as well as the masses of humanity he so dearly loved. His following words reflect his respect for all religions and all of humanity:

> *I consider myself a Hindu, Christian, Muslim,*
> *Jew, Buddhist and Confucian.*

I was a child when I first read these words and was so moved by the simple yet powerful message that it is still in my heart, my mind, and my soul.

I have always been uncomfortable about religion, especially the certainties expressed by many people associated with organized religion. Rejecting their certainties, I rely instead on my instincts when it comes to spiritual matters. This may explain why my religious beliefs are vague and filled with inconsistencies. Nevertheless they have played a major role in forming my prism, but so have my family, especially my father, wife and two of my five grandchildren.

Our Father

On March 9, 2006, my father died after living a full life for ninety-one years. I always called my father "Pop" which is why I am honored that all my grandchildren call me Pop Pop. Noah, my four-year-old grandson, frequently makes cards and drawings for me that he addresses to *Popop*. In spite of the incorrect spelling, I cherish every one he gives me.

When talking with my sister Rosie about Pop, she frequently referred to him as *"Our Father."* This was particularly amusing because all family members knew he did not attend church and he did not believe in God, at least not the God worshipped by any organized religion. A few days prior to his death my daughter Suzy asked him if he believed in God. Firmly but politely he said *"no."* When it was clear that his time was near, Rosie asked if she could *"join a church in his name"* so that he could receive a Christian burial. He agreed because he knew she would experience great pain and guilt if he was not *"buried properly."* I am certain he agreed somewhat reluctantly. Given the opportunity, Rosie gave Pop more than any of us expected; *Pop was buried with the benefit of every possible Christian ritual.*

It would be easy to conclude that my father was an atheist, but I am not sure that is correct because on many levels my father and I agreed about religion, and I am certainly not an atheist. I have doubts about the existence of God, but I suspect that many people of God have doubts.

My father and I spent countless hours enjoying nature during our many fishing trips to Canada, vacation trips with my wife and two daughters, and numerous trips to a lake house in Northern Pennsylvania, which Jean and I owned until four years ago. On several occasions, while we were sitting quietly and enjoying the wonders of nature, Pop would interrupt the silence and say, *"This is my church."* He would pause, look at me and ask, *"Why do you need to attend church, nature is my church?"* I never responded, but I knew exactly what he meant. How could an atheist indicate that *"nature"* was his church? But there is more. When he was frustrated my father would shout *"Dear God"* or *"Dear Lord."* Some would argue that many people use such phrases and that a few words do not provide a true indication of a person's religious beliefs. But I knew my father, and he was a person of few words and he used those words to communicate very clearly. As I indicated earlier, I see uncertainty and contradictions in the religious views of others, and this includes my father.

For many years I was concerned my father would find himself in serious trouble for ignoring rules *(including laws)*, especially those related to hunting and fishing. One day I realized he would not change. Why should he change? When he was found ignoring rules, especially hunting and fishing laws, he was always able to *"talk his way out of trouble."* He did this on more than one occasion when a Pennsylvania game and wildlife officer found him doing something *"questionable."* Having failed to convince my father that he should *"follow the rules"* like everybody else, I simply ignored his behavior and began to call him *"the world's oldest teenager."*

My father would never do anything to harm someone nor would he do anything that was criminal in nature; he simply did things his way. I must admit that some of that has *"rubbed off on me."* My father was a good person, always willing to help friends and family, but he was also one of those unforgettable characters you often hear of but rarely meet. I loved my father and I will miss him, even as I continue to celebrate his life.

My Wife

My wife Jean was born in West Hazleton, Pennsylvania on April 24, 1943. I was born on March 11 of the same year, which means I am approximately six weeks older than she, something she delights in mentioning. Jean graduated from West Hazleton High School in 1961, and I graduated one year earlier from Hazleton High School.

Jean's parents, Claire and John Lindeman, were very nice people and I remember meeting them when Jean and I started dating. Jean has one sibling, her younger sister Sally. I remember Sally as a *"wacky kid"* who was always having fun, behaving strangely, and getting into trouble. She has not changed much, except today she is fifty-nine.

I met Jean the spring of my high school junior year. We were both sixteen and she was a high school sophomore. We started dating and soon discovered we liked each other. In the following year we *"went steady"* and *"broke up"* several times. We were too young to make permanent commitments to each other, but I told her that we would one day be married. I'm sure she thought I was crazy!

At the end of my senior year she escorted me to the Hazleton High School prom. The next year I was her date at the West Hazleton High School prom. By then, I had completed my first year at The Pennsylvania State University (PENN STATE), and everyone knows high school girls love to date college men. We dated many times during the next three years, and we grew closer with each passing day.

I received a B.S. degree in Electrical Engineering in June of 1964 and immediately started working for Bethlehem Steel Corporation. I proposed marriage on Christmas Eve of 1964 and we married on November 27, 1965. In August 1965 I left Bethlehem Steel Corporation and began my teaching career as an instructor at my alma mater, PENN STATE.

I had a full time teaching position with a major university at the tender age of twenty-two. After I signed a one year contract, the Assistant Dean of Engineering commented: *"Your salary is so low that you can be sure of receiving good raises the next couple of years."* He was true to his word, and my salary increased dramatically in a relatively short time.

Our wedding day plans rested on the hope our relatives would be generous. They were, and we paid for our reception with money we received as wedding presents. The first few years of our marriage were financially difficult, but Jean was always upbeat and supported all my career decisions. She was always a joy to be with, and she was a *"peacemaker,"* much like my father.

Prior to our marriage, Jean and I purchased a new fifty-foot trailer. We simply could not afford an apartment. In fact, it was difficult for us to make payments on the trailer. And so, we lived in a trailer park the first three years of our marriage.

Jean's mother died suddenly approximately two years after we married. Her father died almost twenty-eight years ago, the day before our 13th wedding anniversary. Two days later, my mother died. Shortly after we buried our parents, Jean said I was lucky because I still had my father. I told her Pop was also her father, and he confirmed this when he said she was *"just like his daughter."* My wife and my father had a wonderful relationship and in the more than forty years they knew each other, there was never an angry or a hurtful word between them. They had only words of joy and respect for each other.

When Jean was in high school, her nickname was *Jinka*, and to this day many of her friends and some family members still refer to her by that name. Jean was always very popular. But she is more than a nice person with a great smile; she is also intelligent and ambitious. I finished my education in 1975 and since both our daughters were in school, Jean began working and taking college courses. By the time she retired in 2003, she had earned associate, bachelor, and master degrees. She also completed sixty credits beyond the degrees she earned. She started her career as a teacher's aide and become a teacher a few years later. The last ten years of her career were spent as an administrator, reaching the level of Director of Special Education. *Throughout her career she taught, loved, and fought for children who needed help the most: children in special education. Jean is only five feet tall and since I am more than a foot taller, we must seem an odd match to some people. But Jean's heart is bigger than her small stature would suggest ... and so is her courage.*

Jean landed a permanent teaching job a few months after receiving her bachelor's degree. The rest of the credits she earned while working full time. Most of the courses she completed were taught at sites located between forty and eighty miles from our home. I spent many nights at home waiting anxiously for Jean to return from class.

Frequently she drove to and from class over snow covered roads that curved up and down several treacherous mountains. On one occasion I was at home when a severe snow storm arrived while Jean was in class nearly sixty miles away. I had the only four-wheel-drive vehicle in the family, and I was sitting safely at home waiting for Jean to arrive or for her to call me for assistance. Suddenly the phone rang, but it was not Jean. It was our daughter Suzy calling. Suzy was employed as an engineer with a firm near Harrisburg, Pennsylvania. After leaving an evening meeting with a client, she slid off the road and was forced to walk back to the nearest home. She was crying as she asked me to come for her in an area approximately forty miles from where I was located. I had never heard of the small town she was in and I had never been on the road she was referring to. It took ninety minutes of driving over icy roads to reach Suzy. We drove back to our home in Pottsville rather than to her apartment. When we arrived, I was delighted to see Jean patiently waiting for us.

I was frequently concerned for Jean's safety when she drove during winter months, because roads can become dangerous very quickly when temperatures are low. Rain often freezes on roads during winter, and even a small amount of snow can produce slippery conditions. When winter weather threatened to make driving dangerous, I would tell Jean to call in sick or take a vacation day. She always ignored my advice and in frustration I would say, *"You are not the President of the United States. Things will go on without you."*

It took courage for Jean to complete her education and to fight for special needs children. But that pales in comparison to what she did the last two years. If cancer is discovered early, it is possible for the patient to complete the necessary treatments with little or no difficulty. However, I know of several people, including one of my uncles, who choose to die rather than face the pain of chemotherapy or radiation treatments. Jean's cancer was advanced and she endured twelve chemotherapy treatments over a one year period and I watched her suffer. Many people, including Jean, bravely fight cancer with the help of skilled, compassionate medical professionals. Those who fight cancer are my heroes, and those who assist them deserve a special place in heaven.

Daniel Arthur

I always wanted a son, but after having two healthy, beautiful daughters; Jean and I felt our family was complete. On

December 9, 1995 our first grandchild was born. He was a big healthy boy. I was delighted that my daughter Lisa and her husband *(big Dan)*, named their son after his father and me.

Daniel is only ten-years-old, but he is 150 pounds and well over five feet tall. He is healthy and loves playing football and wrestling—both of which he does quite well. Recently he started playing baseball. In a year or so he will be hitting the ball out of the park! Since Daniel was four-years-old, I have talked with him about the importance of having a good mind, good body, and a good heart. I don't take any credit for the way things have turned out, but Daniel has all three. I could write volumes about Daniel's athletic accomplishments and somewhat less about his academic achievements. *Instead I will describe his "heart."*

Daniel is a sensitive kid who cares deeply about all the people around him, especially older family members and others who need assistance or protection. Prior to my father's memorial service, there was a family gathering at the funeral home. Daniel wanted to pay his final respects to my father, but I knew it would be difficult for him. Shortly after Daniel arrived at the funeral home with his parents and sister, I escorted him to my father's coffin holding his left arm with my left hand and placing my right arm across his back.

He stared at my father's face while biting into his bottom lip. I repeatedly told him *"it is okay to cry."* Suddenly he could hold back the tears no longer as grief took control of his entire body. We stayed at the coffin for only a few more moments because other family members were waiting. I took Daniel to the rear of the room where he was able to compose himself with the help of his mother. Soon we left the funeral home and traveled to the church for the memorial mass. Daniel once again broke down and wept uncontrollably. His mother took him to the rear of the church where she again tried to calm him.

Later that day and several times since then, Daniel asked my age and some general questions about my health. I always responded by telling him *"I am healthy"* and *"I will be around for a long time."* At this point I tried to add some humor. If Daniel were an adult I would tell him *"only the good die young, so I will live a very long time."* However, Daniel was too fragile emotionally for any reference to death and he would take that saying literally, raising additional questions in his mind—questions I would not be able to answer. With this in mind, I told Daniel not to worry because *"I will dance at your wedding."* After a short pause, I added *"You must name your first son after me."* As I expected, this brought a smile to Daniel's face. I put my arms around him and kissed him. I was raised believing that males should not hug or kiss, but I hug and kiss all my grandchildren including *"the guys,"* Daniel and Noah.

I have three sisters and no brothers, and two daughters and no sons. I love all my grandchildren equally, but Daniel arrived first and he was the male child I wanted to have in my life since the time Jean and I married more than forty years ago. I thank God for all my grandchildren, but I thank God twice for Daniel.

Lucas Anthony

My daughter Suzanne (*I always called her Suzy*) and John Fredericks married on May 11, 1996. Suzy was twenty-seven and she said her *"biological clock was ticking,"* so they tried to have a child a short time after their marriage. They had some initial difficulties, but these were overcome with the use of medical technology. And so, during the summer of 1999 we received the wonderful news: Suzy was pregnant! However, the joy was not to last. It was Friday, January 13, 2000 and I was at work (*yes, Friday the 13th!*) when I received a telephone call from the receptionist at her doctor's office. Suzy was there for a routine six month pregnancy check up. The message was simple: *"Come to the office as soon as possible because Suzy needs your support!"* In a short time I was sitting in her doctor's office with my two arms wrapped around Suzy. She was crying hysterically. The doctor was visibly distraught and he had tears in his eyes. He could barely speak, but finally he was able to tell me the terrible news. Suzy's baby had polycystic kidneys. This meant that if the baby was born alive, he would die shortly after birth. The doctor's best estimate was *"Suzy will go full term and the baby will be born alive. However, he will die in less than two hours."* I remember thinking how difficult this must be for the doctor, but quickly my attention turned to Suzy. This was the worst moment in my entire life, and yet I knew it was far worse for Suzy. And so, I kept my composure and did my best to comfort her.

From the day we received the terrible news until the day Lucas arrived, John's family and our family rallied around Suzy. Suzy also found comfort and support from friends, especially a nurse she came to know while she was working at the Blue Mountain School District. Looking at the calendar and counting days and months the way pregnant women and their doctors often do, we prayed Lucas would be born on Saint Patrick's Day. Suzy, John, family members, friends and members of several church congregations prayed for Lucas, hoping for a miracle. *God denied all the requests that were made except one:*

Lucas was born on Saint Patrick's Day, March 17, 2000.

Because they knew his life on earth would be short, Suzy and John decided in advance they would share their son only with God. Lucas was baptized by a Roman Catholic priest as I sat next to the door leading into Suzy's hospital room. *I believe I heard Lucas cry, but only once. That was my only connection with Lucas while he was alive. Lucas lived for only sixty-three minutes.* After Lucas died, family members were given the opportunity to hold him. I remember John handing me his son's body, neatly wrapped the way newborn babies are usually prepared. John was crying and he said a few words I can not recall as he handed me the body of my grandson. I still have a clear image of my grandson's beautiful face and during moments of solitude, I can still feel him in my arms.

Shortly after Lucas was buried, Suzy and John considered the possibility of having another baby. Privately Jean and I hoped they would not try, but we were careful not to influence their decision. We told them we would support any decision they made. They tried again and Noah was born on May 1, 2001, approximately thirteen months after Lucas died. Another effort, again supported by medical technology, produced Helena. She was born on February 25, 2004. The joy of seeing Suzy and John bring two beautiful, healthy children into the world did much to cure the pain we all felt just a short time earlier.

The death of Lucas made our families appreciate the joys of life, which we frequently take for granted. In addition, Suzy and John are better people and better parents than they would have been in the absence of Lucas. I have great pride in Suzy and John, for they handled a devastating period in their lives with honor and unbelievable courage.

It is March 17, 2006 and I am sitting on my favorite beach in South Carolina. If he had survived, Lucas would be six-years-old today. This is the day I set aside to write about Lucas. I think of Lucas often, but on Saint Patrick's Day it is different because this is his day. Although he died six years ago, Lucas is always with me. For reasons that are unknown to me, I feel guilty about his death. Perhaps my guilt is the way I keep his spirit alive within me. Even now, I can not write these words without weeping, for I love and deeply miss the grandson I never knew.

When I think of my four surviving grandchildren, my heart is filled with joy and I smile or even laugh. I share my feelings about Lucas with my wife and my daughter Lisa, but I do not weep in their presence, for I choose to mourn alone. Tonight I will call my daughter Suzy and her husband John. We will not discuss Lucas directly. It would be too painful for us. But they will know it is my way of connecting with them and Lucas.

A grandchild who lived only sixty-three minutes has had a profound effect on all that I am. His passing made me a better person and demonstrated the importance of family. His death also had an enormous effect on Suzy and John. Today they adore their children in a way that only parents who have lost a child could ever understand.

The death or suffering of a loved one creates connections in the mind with other loved ones who have died or suffered. My mind frequently jumps from Lucas to my father's life and death, to my wife's ongoing battle with cancer. This always happens in church when the minister or priest asks the congregation to pray silently for loved ones who have passed or who are suffering. I think of Pop, Lucas, and my wife in an instant. I am incapable of doing anything else. At times I compare my father's long, rich life that seems complete to me and the short time Lucas had with a family that adored him. *I am not able to accept what happened to Lucas—but I know I must.*

When I think of my wife and the difficult journey she has had the last two years, I face the possibility her life could end long before it should. *Oh God, I pray that does not happen!* I was unable to help Lucas. I am his grandfather, I should have been able to help him, but I never did! Will I one day look back on the passing of my precious wife and curse my inability to help her? I try to help her, but it seems her destiny is in the hands of God. *No, here I must express it my way—her destiny is with a Greater Presence.*

Although this book is far from complete, writing it, especially this section, has helped me deal with the loss of Lucas. Before starting to write this book, I could not write the following words and I still can not speak them:

Lucas is with me now and will be until the day I die. I hope there is a God and life after death because when I cross the river for the last time, I will think of family. And if there is life after death, I will look for Lucas when I arrive on the other side, for I miss him terribly.

Part Two

Two Difficult Years

The time between Jean's 61st and 63rd birthdays was very difficult for Jean and our entire family. What follows in this portion of the book is a "Journey of The Mind" in combination with a chronology of medical and personal events that has taken place during these two years. Data presented is taken from the following sources:

1. Jean's personal planners for 2004, 2005, and 2006.
2. My personal planners for the same years.
3. A journal Jean kept from December 2004 to March 2005. (She was not able to maintain a journal after March 2005.)
4. Jean's medical records.
5. Our financial and insurance records.
6. Our recollections of events.
7. Discussions with family members.

It is impossible to forget events of the last two years including the emotions we all experienced. The emotions were connected to specific events, especially medical events so linking the two was relatively easy. *While Jean's drama was unfolding, the downward spiral of my father's life was taking place, ending with his death on March 9, 2006.*

Jean's medical chronicle took place in an environment filled with fear, but also with hope. Events of the last two years produced significant successes, but there remains cause for continued anxiety. In contrast, my father's situation had an obvious inevitability about it. Advanced age, steadily declining physical mobility, and an increasing array of medical problems meant my father's time was limited. Recognizing this, family members did everything possible to care for my father and to *"celebrate"* with him until his end came.

CHAPTER 3

Pancreatitis and Medical Tests
April to September 2004

It has been many years since Jean enjoyed celebrating her birthday with a traditional party involving family and friends. So when I asked how we would celebrate her 61st birthday, I was not surprised when she said she did not want a party and did not want to celebrate. I approached her at least a month before her birthday hoping she would agree to a special birthday vacation trip, but even this idea was rejected. Finally I came up with an idea she could not reject. I frequently talk to Tim Holden while working out at a fitness center in Minersville, Pennsylvania. Tim is the Democratic congressman from the 17th District of Pennsylvania. Although we are both Republicans, Jean and I always voted for Tim because he is conservative, honest, and a *"good guy."*

Several years earlier, Tim ran for Schuylkill County Sheriff and Jean and I held a *"meet the candidate"* party for him. The party was not a fundraiser, just an opportunity for our mostly Republican friends to meet Tim. In view of this, I knew Jean would be receptive to having another *"meet Tim Holden party,"* especially if I did most of the work organizing and hosting the party. Oh yes, the party had to be up to Jean's standards. She said, *"No ring bologna and beer party."* I was confident the best time for the party would be on or near Jean's birthday. Working with Tim's campaign staff, we selected the best time for Tim that also matched our schedule, especially our travel plans. Jean and I frequently traveled to South Carolina, and she would never agree to change our travel plans for something as insignificant as a birthday party. Therefore I was pleasantly surprised that Jean accepted her birthday, April 24, 2004, as the date for the party.

Jean suggested we have a wine and cheese party and have a caterer supply and serve hors d'œuvres. She also helped me with the guest list. I was very happy with the way things were coming together: assisting Tim Holden in his bid for reelection; a party on Jean's birthday; and bringing friends together, some of whom we had not seen in over a year.

I remember inviting Joan and Tom. I spoke with Joan by telephone and invited her and her husband Tom. *She paused and then said, "Artie, do you know Tom has Alzheimer's?" My response was short but sincere, "I don't give a damn, Tom's my friend and I would like to see him at the party."* I went on to say they would know everyone at the party and identified many people they knew who were coming. Finally Joan agreed to come and said she would bring Tom. Then Joan asked if she could make a cake or some dessert for the party. I told her *"no."* She had plenty to do taking care of Tom.

Later, I told Jean about my discussion with Joan. We had heard Tom had Alzheimer's, but I held out hope it was merely a rumor. One reason I remember my conversation with Joan so clearly is because she offered to make a cake for the party and I loved her cooking, especially the wonderful desserts she made! It was also incredibly nice of her to make the offer when it was clear she had her hands full taking care of Tom.

The day of the party arrived and everything was coming together beautifully. The house was cleaned and organized for the party. The enclosed patio and yard area were all ready. Cheese was cut, wine was chilled, paper products were all in place, and the caterer had arrived early as planned. The door bell rang and the first guests arrived. They knew their way around the house, so I told them to come in, get a drink, and have something to eat.

As soon as the first guests arrived, Jean said she was sick. She then went to our ground floor bathroom and began to vomit. At this point I was focused on the party and the forty to fifty guests who were about to arrive. For a few minutes I was simply overwhelmed. Guests were arriving, the caterer was asking questions, and my wife was kneeling next to the toilet. With great difficulty, Jean told me to continue with the party. She told me she was having another stomach virus attack, and she would be fine.

Jean had a stomach virus at least five times in the previous year, including an episode when she was at a conference in the Pocono Mountains of Pennsylvania. On that occasion, she was taken to a hospital emergency room for medical care. Another time we were in South Carolina for a nine or ten day trip and she became sick twice! The symptoms of what we thought were bouts of stomach virus were always the same: sudden onset of vomiting and diarrhea, and at times, pain in her stomach. Since Jean identified her illness as a stomach virus, I was confident she would recover quickly as she had in the past.

So the party continued, although the congressman and others offered to terminate the event. I declined their offer thinking this had happened in the past, and Jean's illness was not serious. In view of Jean's condition, it was amazing how well the party went. Two of our friends, Margie and Fran, spent most of their evening caring for Jean. Margie is Jean's best friend whom we half jokingly refer to as a *"Saint"* because she cares for so many friends and family members, even when she is experiencing great pain and discomfort. Patti, another of our wonderful friends, helped me with food, drinks, and other chores Jean would have normally done. I would have been lost without the help of these three long time friends.

In spite of Jean's illness, there were a few moments of joy that night. When Joan and Tom came to the door I was pleasantly surprised by Tom. His speech was a bit slow, but he recognized me immediately, extending his hand to shake the same way we had done many times in the past. I also had a brief but pleasant conversation with Patti's husband John. He was interested in hearing about our place in Myrtle Beach, South Carolina. We had just sold our two bedroom condo and purchased a three bedroom condo, both in the same building. The sale of the two bedroom unit was complete, but the closing on the purchase of the three bedroom unit was scheduled for the week after the party. Near the end of our conversation, John told me to call him if I came across any good properties. He said he would be interested in buying a vacation property in South Carolina, and he trusted my judgment. I made a mental note of his interest.

Life has many surprises in store for us and a painful irony was about to reveal itself. A few months after the party, a very nice place became available just a short distance from our condo, so I made an attempt to reach John. My efforts were unsuccessful because his wife Patti had developed a serious illness with no known cure. Ironically, Patti was one of the three women who helped me the night of the party when Jean became ill. For most of the last two years, John has focused on his wife's declining health. Jean and I often speak of them and pray for them. I wish I could help John and Patti in some way.

The party went on as planned and ended as scheduled. Everyone thanked me for inviting them to the party and expressed concern for Jean. I assured them she would be fine; this was simply a repeat of a stomach virus she had in the past. Margie and Patti helped me clean up the house and Jean went upstairs to a bedroom. We called Jean's sister Sally, a registered nurse with thirty years of experience, for some medical advice as we had done many times in the past. Sally said we should wait an hour or so to see if Jean's condition improved, adding I should take Jean to the emergency room of the hospital if her condition became more serious. Jean seemed to improve, so I tried to get some sleep.

Later that evening, I believe it was around 11 pm, Jean was in terrible pain and she woke me saying she needed to get to the hospital immediately. Then she became angry with me because she said I was taking too much time dressing. By the time we arrived at the hospital, her anger increased and she demanded I drop her off at the emergency room door and leave. I agreed with her, parked the car, and walked back to the emergency room. I had learned to agree with her and then do what I thought was best. I entered the hospital and was directed to the room where she was already in a bed and dressed in a hospital robe. She again became angry and demanded that I go home. I agreed and went to the waiting room. A few minutes later a nurse came for me and said my wife wanted me to return.

Jean was calm now and I knew medications were already being given to her. Within minutes a doctor appeared and told us a blood sample would be taken so that her condition could be evaluated. I expected the results of the *"blood work"* would not be available for several days, but he said the results would be back within an hour. He was correct. *In less than an hour the doctor returned to tell us Jean had pancreatitis. This was the start of my education in medical terms and concepts, an education which continues to this day.* I had heard of pancreatitis, but I knew nothing about its causes, symptoms, treatment, or dangers. The doctor told us that Jean would be admitted to the hospital, and she would begin to receive medications. He said the pancreatitis was probably caused by gall stones, and she would be fine.

After Jean was admitted and taken to her hospital room, I left and went home. The next morning I called our daughters, Sally, and my sister Rosie to inform them of the previous night's events. A short time later I arrived at the hospital. Jean was resting peacefully and as expected, she was receiving medications. I remember she was receiving fluids intravenously. I am not sure how or why he was assigned to Jean, but Doctor Franklin became her attending physician.

Doctor Franklin told us that pancreatitis was usually caused by gall stones or excessive consumption of alcohol over a long period of time. Then he added that 10% of the time the cause is unknown. This was confirmed by reading material my daughter Lisa gave me a short time later. He went on to say he expected gall stones were the cause in Jean's case. However, later that day we learned the medical tests produced no evidence Jean had gall stones.

Jean was no longer in pain and additional blood work revealed the liver enzymes used to mark or diagnose pancreatitis were falling. This was good news because it meant Jean would recover, and in a few days she would be released from the hospital. It also meant that she would not require surgery for removal of gall stones. On April 26, Jean's second full day in the hospital, Dr. Martino, a family friend, paid her a social visit while he made his visitation rounds in the hospital. He had heard Jean was in the hospital for pancreatitis. When entering the room he said, *"Don't worry I'll remove your gall stones and you will be out of here in no time."* I told him the necessary tests were performed, and they indicated Jean did not have gall stones. He looked puzzled and was uncharacteristically quiet for a few moments. He then became very serious and pointing his finger at Jean he told her she should never have another drink of alcohol; none for the rest of her life. I remember all of this very clearly because of what happened next. I asked Dr. Martino if a person could die from pancreatitis. He said yes and then identified someone we knew who died after their second pancreatitis attack. I assumed pancreatitis could result in death, but I wanted to be certain. I also wanted Jean to know the seriousness of her condition.

Like many people, Jean drank wine and occasionally beer. She usually drank red wine, believing it to be part of the so-called Mediterranean Diet, which according to some medical experts, helps reduce the chances of developing heart disease. Jean's mother died from a heart attack and her sister Sally had suffered a heart attack. For years Jean told me her mother died at age fifty and she expected to die from a heart attack when she reached that age. *Jean is now sixty-three.* The point is she focused her efforts on preventing heart disease. Regular exercise, a wide range of supplements, weight control, and red wine were her main weapons in the private war she waged against possible heart disease. Jean often cited what she believed to be solid scientific evidence supporting her decisions to take numerous supplements and to drink red wine. We often had minor disagreements about her use of supplements and more serious arguments about the benefits of drinking red wine. Jean was convinced alcohol was not the cause of her pancreatitis attack and so she and Dr. Franklin explored other possible causes focusing on medications she took. Several months earlier, Jean developed herpes simplex in her right eye. This was a serious problem that could have resulted in the loss of vision in that eye.

The medication prescribed for her worked well, and she was still taking it when she entered the hospital. Hearing this, Dr. Franklin told her to discontinue the use of this medication until he had a chance to evaluate it. Before she left the hospital, he informed her the medication did not cause her pancreatitis and she should resume taking it.

Jean spent seven nights in the hospital and was tired and emotionally drained when she came home. She recovered in a few days and we traveled to South Carolina for a well deserved vacation. We were both shaken by what had happened to her, but we had different opinions as to the cause of the pancreatitis attack as well as the measures that should be taken to prevent a reoccurrence. However, Jean agreed to discontinue consumption of all alcoholic beverages. When we arrived in South Carolina, I bought several bottles of non-alcoholic wine. She tried it but did not like it. However, we discovered she liked non-alcoholic beer. I rarely drank alcoholic beverages, so it was surprising I also liked it.

The realization that Jean could have died from the first pancreatitis attack, and could possibly die if there was a second attack, had a profound effect on me and although she didn't say it, I believe it had a similar impact on Jean. For the first time in my life I realized that she could die in the not too distant future. It did not take long to expand my thinking and realize I too could die in the next few years because like Jean, I had also passed my 60th birthday and was beginning to develop a wide range of ailments.

As happened so many times these past two years, an event in the present triggered a vivid image of the past. One image from the past came to mind as soon as I realized Jean could have died. *When I was seven years old my maternal grandmother died. She was a devout Greek Catholic who attended mass every morning. She was a small, gentle woman who passed away in church during mass—I still find that amazing.* There is little doubt she died in a place and in a manner that gave her and most of her family enormous comfort. But even a child could see my grandfather did not feel any comfort with the manner in which she died. I don't believe he felt any anger, because anger was never within him, but it was obvious he felt deep pain and sorrow. The wake was held in my grandparent's home, in a small town outside of Hazleton, Pennsylvania. I remember so many details of my grandmother's death because it was the first time I saw a deceased loved one. But what I remember most clearly was my grandfather.

My grandmother's coffin was in the largest open area on the ground floor of their modest home, and my grandfather stood to the right of the coffin wearing a black suit, black tie and white shirt. He was tall, slim and muscular from years of shoveling coal on his job. He was very erect. In fact he looked like a soldier standing at attention. *I remember all of this, but what I remember most was how sad he was. He was not crying and no one spoke to him, perhaps because his profound sorrow filled the room.*

My grandfather died approximately one year after my grand-mother's death. Over the years, I discussed his death with my mother, father, and other family members. Everyone I spoke to agreed: My grandfather died of a broken heart. He simply could not live without his wife. It is easy to see how Jean's pancreatitis attack could evoke this distant memory. To this day I recall the death of my grandmother, the sadness of my grandfather at her passing, and finally his death. I worry that the same fate may await Jean and me. The thought of Jean dying disturbs me deeply, but I do not fear my own death. However, I know the passing of either of us would do great harm to the families of our daughters, especially to our wonderful grandchildren. Our grandchildren would survive and grow to be good people, but the passing of either of us would diminish the quality of their lives, and I would hate to have that happen!

Jean retired from the Schuylkill Intermediate Unit 29, a consortium of school districts, in November 2003, and I had retired from The Pennsylvania State University in December of 2001. We were enjoying the good life we worked so hard for when Jean became ill. Prior to her illness, our lives revolved around frequent trips, especially to South Carolina, enjoying our grandchildren and spending quality time with my father.

A Few Words about Pop

In May of 2004 my father had remarkable mental ability for a man who would turn ninety in two months. There were several simple benchmarks I used to gauge my father's mental and physical well being. Playing cards, playing checkers, and casual conversation were the best ways to determine if he was mentally alert. It was clear that he was slightly forgetful and his speech and thinking were slow and becoming slower. *But he still played cards better than I could and I never beat him at checkers. As far as I was concerned, his mental ability was excellent for a man who was nearly ninety. His physical well being was another matter.*

In 1991, Jean and I bought a beautiful five and one half acre lake front parcel of land in Northern Pennsylvania. The *lake had a wide variety of fish and plenty of them. Even better, the area had few people and an abundance of deer. My father loved the lake and was always ready to spend a few days or even a week there with me.*

Pop spent most winters in Florida with my sister Rosie and her husband Pete. There was one exception. The winter of 1994 was very cold and for some reason my father did not travel to Florida that year. The lake was frozen solid and covered with at least a foot of snow. I was planning a long weekend at the lake house to do some inside work *(trim work, staining and painting)*. As long as I could work at my own pace, the work was enjoyable. On this particular weekend, conditions were ideal for ice fishing, so I asked Pop if he was interested. He said *"yes."* Next I asked Dan, then my daughter's fiancé, if he would be interested in spending an ice fishing weekend at the lake. There was a series of jobs he would be responsible for and I made this very clear to him. His most important job was to *"take care of my father."* My father was in excellent health, but he was seventy-nine years old. In addition, Dan would need to drill the ice fishing holes, by hand of course, shovel snow to make the paths from the house to the lake and from hole to hole. Lastly, it would be his job to carry all the necessary gear to the lake and clean it up at the end of the day. Dan agreed to all of this and it worked out perfectly.

Dan is a big, strong guy who loves nature and fishing, and he had enormous respect for my father. Dan and my father fished while I worked on the inside of the house and did the cooking. Daylight ends early during the winter and the temperature drops drastically even before the sun sets, so Dan and my father were always inside before 5 pm and eating a large meal before 5:30 pm. Cable TV was not available and the antenna was of little value, so we relied on a large library of VCR movies to provide entertainment. I don't know what movies we watched, but it was either a cowboy or war movie because they were the only kind my father was interested in. Besides, Dan and I also enjoyed them. The second day of the trip was wonderful. Dan had already done the hard work, so he and my father simply waited for the sun to warm things up and then they started their second day of ice fishing. Before too long Dan asked me for the key to the shed. He took two patio lounge chairs from the shed and carried them to the lake so that the two of them could be comfortable while they fished. I'm sure it was not Dan's idea. It was the middle of winter and everything was covered by a thick layer of snow. Yet the sun was bright, the air was clear and surprisingly, it was so warm that it felt like a spring day.

About 1 or 2 in the afternoon I walked to the lake to see how the fishing was going and to enjoy the unusual weather. My father was asleep in his lounge chair, facing the sun as if he were sunbathing. It was so warm he had removed his coat. Dan took an ice chest from the shed so my father could extend his legs and use it as a foot stool. In spite of their leisurely approach to ice fishing, they caught a few fish including one very large bass my father caught. It was absolutely a perfect weekend of ice fishing.

My father's physical and mental abilities were exceptional for someone who was nearly eighty. When the weather was mild, my father had no difficulty walking two to four miles with me, without the benefit of a cane or walking stick. He was a better card player than me and I never beat him in checkers, one of his favorite activities. In addition, he was not on any medications and rarely saw a doctor!

My father had a few more years of near perfect health—it is impossible to determine when his physical ability began to decline—but I believe it was about eight years ago when he was eighty-four. He could not walk as far or as often as he once did, and he began to use a walking stick. He also slept more. He took frequent naps and would sleep much longer in the morning. By the time he was eighty-six, his mobility had declined so drastically he could no longer join me when I traveled to the lake. He could not climb the steps inside the house or the porch steps leading into the house. He also lacked the strength and coordination to fish.

I had enjoyed nature all my life with my father at my side, but sadly this source of joy was now denied to both of us.

Age had finally begun to take its toll on my father, and I was not spared the physical problems that come with senior citizen status. I had increased pain in my right ankle and left knee and with each passing year I found the cold winter months at the lake increasingly difficult. Since I was the only person in the family willing to visit the lake house in winter, it became obvious that Jean and I needed to sell this wonderful place where Pop and I had spent so many memorable times. After some initial hesitation, Jean agreed. We sold the lake house in the spring of 2002 and *"rolled the money over"* to buy a condo in Myrtle Beach, South Carolina. One happy chapter of our lives ended and another began. That same year my father moved in with my sister Rosie and her husband Pete. It was impossible for him to enter or exit the home where he and my mother raised my three sisters and me. The steps leading into the front of the house and those in the rear of the house were far more than he could handle without assistance from at least two adults. Even Rosie's house and the home Jean and I lived in presented obstacles—steps to climb and bathrooms that were not handicap friendly.

In May of 2004, less than two weeks after Jean experienced pancreatitis, my father moved into an assisted living facility in Hazleton, Pennsylvania—*The Laurels Senior Retirement Center*—and he was not happy about it! Someone had to be with him—or at least available—at all times to help with his bathroom needs and to administer the many medications he now relied on. Rosie and Pete had given so much of their lives to caring for others, but they could no longer provide the care my father needed.

The entire family knew it was time for my father to move into a facility organized to satisfy the specific needs of senior citizens—a place where he could be constantly monitored and would have the frequent human contact that he so needed and enjoyed. But this was a very sad, irreversible step in my father's long life and there was deep sorrow and concern throughout the family. In spite of my father's dissatisfaction with his new home, everyone tried to be positive—especially when communicating with him. After a few weeks, my father made friends and found he could still have daily contact with family members. Gradually he accepted the reality of his new life. He simply created a circle of happiness in a new location—family, old friends, new friends—everything properly organized so my father could continue living a good life.

My father was never interested in money or possessions. His greatest joys all included being in contact with friends and family. He loved talking, playing cards, and eating with people. He never tired of these things. Rosie was the center of his world before and after he became a resident of the Laurels—but now she had the Laurels as a constant stabilizing force in my father's life. Because he was at the Laurels, it was much easier for Rosie to coordinate the comings and goings of the many friends and family who wanted to continue experiencing the joy he so eagerly offered. For my part, I tried to visit at least once a week for two or three hours. Pop and I would go out for lunch or dinner and if he was strong enough and the weather was mild, we would shop at the local mall. *Frequently Jean would join us. These were special visits because Pop loved to talk and joke with her.*

Shortly after he entered The Laurels, Rosie and I began to plan our father's 90th birthday celebration. His birth date was July 11, but the celebration was held on July 24, 2004. Ten years earlier, his 80th birthday was a major celebration in the Marsicano family and it was held at a neighborhood bar which was previously owned by my father's brothers. (*It was Marsicano's Bar and Grill when my uncles owned and operated it.*) We considered having his 90th birthday party at the same location, but this idea did not remain under consideration for very long because my father and other elderly family members would not be able to complete the long walk from their cars to the dining area. They would also have great difficulty in the bathrooms, which were not designed for people with disabilities. Suddenly, we decided on the obvious: the party was held where my father lived, at the Laurels. We would have the meal catered (*Italian food of course*) and hire an entertainer for the day—one who could sing the Italian songs my father loved. This also made it easy to invite the staff and residents of the Laurels.

The party was a huge success, attended by more than fifty friends and family members. In addition, many residents and employees of The Laurels attended. The food was prepared by Casamato's Ristorante and it was wonderful. There was even a strolling performer who sang a wide range of Italian songs while playing a guitar. For several weeks after the party we continued to relive the event, especially after the photographs were developed. *It is almost two years after the party, and I still enjoy looking at the fifty or sixty wonderful photographs in our 2004 family album. My favorite is a picture of Jean standing next to my father while he supports himself with his walker.*

Returning to the Two Year Period in Jean's Life

Jean looked so happy and healthy on this photograph and on another standing next to me. She had every reason to be happy. She had recovered from her illness and on May 4 we closed on the purchase of a three bedroom/three bathroom condo in Myrtle Beach, South Carolina. Oh yes, we had a fantastic view of the ocean. By the end of the month we had purchased new furniture to replace most of the furniture that was included with the condo purchase and we had hired contractors to make several large improvements.

The good news continued after we returned from South Carolina at the end of May. On June 2, Jean visited her gynecologist for a PAP test and pelvic internal—*a total female physical*—and she was given a positive report. On June 3 she had a CT scan as part of the continuing evaluation related to her April 24 pancreatitis attack. On June 9 during the follow up appointment with Dr. Franklin, she again received good news. The CT scan found nothing abnormal. However, the CT scan did not include her reproductive organs. Jean also had several significant eye problems resulting in a cornea evaluation on June 4. Her eye doctor reassured her but suggested she see an additional eye specialist in September.

Jean had completed medical evaluations during June 2004 for three totally unrelated *"medical issues"* and received nothing but positive results. The news was so uplifting that we decided to *"take a vacation"* as a way to celebrate—and what could be better than to take a trip with our sisters Rosie and Sally? They agreed to come and the trip was scheduled for early August. For more than twenty-five years I had traveled to Canada every summer with my father for a one or two week fishing trip. These were wonderful times, but it had been a long time since my father could make such a trip. Approximately ten years earlier I began to invite other family members and friends to join me for summer vacations in Canada. I missed having my father with me on these trips—it actually felt *"strange"* the first few times I traveled north without him. My father never expressed any regrets about my traveling without him, and he enjoyed the stories and photographs I brought back with me. Of course I always brought back a hat, tee shirt or sweat shirt for him.

Because I had so many wonderful experiences in Canada, it was easy for me to plan a seven day trip there which Rosie, Sally, my wife and I would enjoy. Naturally, I was the driver and the general purpose … *man Friday*. We spent four nights in a two bedroom suite in Ottawa, the capital of Canada, followed by three nights in a suite in Toronto: Canada's largest city.

Once in Ottawa, it was an easy walk to the river that separates the English speaking province of Ontario and the French speaking province of Quebec. I was intrigued by this and enjoyed walking from the English side of the river to the French side— something I did every day! I love experiencing different cultures, so this was very special for me. We heard there was a large casino on the French side of the river and soon realized it could be seen from our hotel. So the day after we arrived, we decided to take a leisurely walk to the casino. What a mistake! We discovered *"you can't get there from here"* can be a reality. We walked for several hours trying to get to the casino. We could see it, but we could not find a road or a street that would take us there! There was always a river, lake or forest blocking us. After walking for three hours we finally got close to the casino with only one small lake between us and hours of gambling. We found a path around the lake and in a short time we were in the casino. We were hungry, thirsty, dirty, and very tired, but we had survived our first surprise of the trip. There were more to follow.

Shared stress can produce strong bonds, and so *"the girls"* began calling themselves the McGuire Sisters, a vocal group from the 1940s. Later that day, they began to call me Dean Martin. I responded by saying, *"Dean Martin did not make any movies with The Three Stooges."* I left the casino before *"the girls"* and took a taxi back to our hotel. We returned to the casino two more times but always by taxi! We spent four fun filled days in Ottawa, and on the fifth day we headed west toward Toronto.

Along the way we found another casino in the middle of nowhere, and of course we stopped for a meal. And since we were already there ... *we gambled!* The casino was located in Gananogue (*We never figured out how to pronounce it.*) on the Canadian side of the Saint Lawrence River. Sally and I lost (*I never win!*), but Rosie and Jean won.

We arrived in Toronto late in the afternoon and spent the rest of the day exploring the area around our hotel. The next day Sally and Rosie toured, shopped, and for a time *"got lost."* Jean and I toured the city and went to the top of the CN Tower. (*I never figured out what CN stood for.*) The view was unbelievable and the tower was so high it was frightening. That evening the four of us went to a play and we enjoyed every minute of it. The next day we took a ferry to Toronto Islands Park. We spent most of our time exploring the park and ended the day still on the island at a quaint, very expensive restaurant. We decided to eat outside. We laughed a lot, even while the insects were biting our legs. We put candles under our table to control the little monsters, but it did not help. We ordered soup with our meal; it was fifteen dollars a bowl and—we laughed because Sally said her husband Dennis would kill her if he knew how much the meal cost. I guess we were a bit crazy because it was the last night of a wonderful vacation.

We returned home the next day and in a short time Jean and I were back into our usual routine—medical visits, traveling to the Laurels to see my father, and enjoying our grandchildren. On August 16 Jean had a stress test—her heart was just fine—followed by a colonoscopy and endoscopy on August 20. Again the results were all good.

My father had adjusted to his life at the Laurels, where he had many friends and the staff was always kind to him. My sister Rosie, Uncle Joe—my father's only surviving sibling—and many family members took turns taking Pop out for a dining experience or for a walk in the Mall. On special occasions Pop would spend the day at Rosie's house or at the home of her son Peter. Occasionally Pop would become difficult and refuse to use his cane or his walker. This was a problem because he could barely walk with the support of a cane, and he needed a walker to help lift himself off the toilet when he used a bathroom that was not designed for disabled people. After a month or so this problem faded as he accepted the reality of his reduced mobility and strength—after that he always used the walker. Even with the walker and physical therapy several times a week, his mobility and strength continued to decline.

Pop's emotional state was rarely influenced by his declining health. The only exception was when he was denied an opportunity to engage in a social activity, especially a family activity, because of his physical limitations. This meant there was a serious problem on the horizon, because Rosie and Pete spent several months in Florida every winter and Pop usually went with them. This year his physical limitations might make it impossible for him to make the trip. During the fall this was left as an *"open question."* Pop never acknowledged he was unable to travel, and Rosie never confirmed he would be traveling to Florida with her and her husband. *In the end Pop got his way—he traveled to Florida with Rosie and Pete that winter, but it was the last time.*

Pop was not the only one with medical problems. On September 29, Jean and I drove to Reading for our annual arthritis evaluations with Dr. Marco. He was also interested in Jean's bone density and concerned about her fibromyalgia: a condition he identified more than ten years earlier. My left knee had advanced arthritis *(bone on bone),* which was my most troublesome medical problem. Arthritis in my right knee, left hip and neck also limited my activities.

As expected, the results of my evaluation resulted in a significant change in my life style and had the potential for significantly reducing our income. Engineering consulting had been a source of personal pride and significant income for more than twenty-five years; but now health problems, especially pain in my left knee, convinced me that I could not continue my consulting work. Kneeling, standing, climbing stairs and ladders were activities I did on a regular basis during my consulting work, but now they produced extreme pain. Surprisingly, walking at moderate speed or riding an exercise bike did not produce knee pain—and both activities helped control my weight and strengthen my legs.

The appointment with Dr. Marco convinced me to end my consulting work as soon as possible. I would try to complete all the consulting work I had previously agreed to; accept no future work; and inform clients I was retiring. I was certain this could be done by the end of the year. Suddenly I realized that on January 1, 2005, I would be totally retired. Jean knew we would have less money to spend in the future, but she supported my decision as she always did.

CHAPTER 4

Ovarian Cancer
October to December 2004

October is my favorite month in South Carolina—fewer tourists, mild weather, remarkably warm ocean, and very light automobile traffic. We spent most of the month in South Carolina, returning to Pennsylvania so I could complete a consulting job I started in August. I spent October 29 at a manufacturing site with Pennsylvania Department of Revenue officials. They wanted to verify some calculations presented in an energy analysis I wrote earlier in the year. Apparently they were satisfied—in a week or so the report was officially approved by the Department. This left one last consulting job, after which I would never again need to *"earn a living."* Jean and I would be satisfied living on our pensions.

By now Jean and I had developed a plan for dividing our time between Pennsylvania and South Carolina. We would spend two or three weeks in South Carolina and travel back to Pennsylvania for the end of the month. Once in Pennsylvania we would take care of our medical needs—doctor visits, medical tests and order prescription drugs—pay bills, visit my father, spend time with our grandchildren, and prepare for the return trip. This is what we planned for November with two significant differences. Tuesday, November 2, 2004 was Election Day and we arrived at the polls very early. We voted, got into our automobile that was packed the night before, and drove to Emporia, Virginia where we had reserved a two room suite with two television sets. We ordered pizza and watched the election returns as we ate. As expected the election returns were exciting. The next day we followed the returns and related news on the radio as we completed the trip to South Carolina. November was another wonderful month and we returned home for our 39th wedding anniversary on November 27. I also had two medical appointments: one relating to a neck and spine problem and the other was my annual prostate examination.

In early December we returned to South Carolina. We hoped to finish remodeling work on the condo and buy additional furniture. On December 8, Jean began to experience pressure in her abdomen. She called Sally for advice and was told, *"It is probably a bladder infection so make an appointment with your gynecologist."*

Jean scheduled the appointment for December 14. This was perfect for me because I planned on traveling to the Philadelphia area that afternoon, spend the night at a hotel and complete my last day of consulting work the next day. At around 6 pm on December 14, I called home as I did every night when I was away on a consulting trip. *Jean answered the telephone and she was hysterical. She had every reason to be upset. She said her gynecologist told her she probably had ovarian cancer! I did not believe it. How could a doctor arrive at such a conclusion in less than one day? It did not make sense! That evening I spent several hours on the tele-*

phone discussing the situation with my daughters, my sister Rosie, and Jean's sister Sally.

The next morning I started my work at the plant very early. I completed my data collection as soon as I could and raced home arriving at approximately 3 pm. An analysis of the data would take place on another day. When I left Jean our lives were happy, stable, and stress free; but in less than twenty-four hours our world *"turned upside down."* Everything had changed. All of our plans and dreams seemed to vanish in an instant. All that mattered was taking care of Jean and hoping it was all a huge mistake we would one day laugh at.

When I arrived home Jean was waiting for me. We hugged and kissed and I began to ask questions and search for answers. There was so much information and so much more I needed to know—it was overwhelming. *My "cancer education" was beginning and my engineering background was of enormous value.*

During the December 14 appointment, Dr. Knight did a pelvic examination and concluded that Jean probably had ovarian cancer. Dr. Knight suggested an ultrasonic imaging test as a way to confirm what she suspected. The test was scheduled for January 3—nearly three weeks later. The technician who did ultrasonic testing for Dr. Knight was about to leave the office and heard Jean complain about the delay. Fortunately, the technician agreed to do the test immediately.

Masses were found on both ovaries (7x6.7cm on the right ovary and 3.9x3.5cm on the left ovary). Before Jean left the office, blood was drawn to test for the "ovarian cancer marker" ... CA125. I did not realize that some cancers have a "marker" found in the blood that may indicate the presence of the cancer and suggest to some extent, the severity of the cancer. As Jean told me all of this, I was initially overcome with all the details, or perhaps it was just the shock of learning Jean could have cancer.

Jean told me she had seen Dr. Swavic, our primary care physician, a short time after receiving the awful news from Dr. Knight. He wisely prescribed medication to deal with her emotional state and cautioned her not to jump to any conclusions after just one test: the ultrasonic imaging—*because medical testing procedures have so many false positives.* The medications helped, but it was impossible to subdue the "racing thoughts," stress and anxiety that were tormenting her.

By the next day we received the ovarian cancer blood marker results. Jean's CA125 was 1006, which was unbelievably high compared with the normal range of 35 or less! That same day (December 15) a CAT scan was performed. Dr. Knight communicated the results to Jean the next day by telephone. The CAT scan was consistent with the CA125 and ultrasonic imaging results. Based upon my reading and results of three different medical tests—I was absolutely certain Jean had ovarian cancer! Now what? What should we do? We felt an enormous sense of urgency, but we also knew significant progress had already been made. Still, we recognized the need to do things wisely, not just quickly!

Jean was in a state of panic. We had to do the right things and do them quickly, otherwise the evil that had invaded her body would kill her! It was that simple. I am usually calm and strong in the midst of a crisis, but not this time. In spite of our extreme anxiety, we both resolved to do our best. Only then would we be able to live with the results. When faced with personal tragedy the best thing to do is connect with family, friends, and God. We did that and it helped.

Margie, Jean's best friend, told us to contact her brother for advice. Her brother was a gynecologist living in Arizona. His nickname suited him perfectly: *Pal.* With the help of friends we had not seen in a few years, our children helped us track down another gynecologist, who was also an oncologist. He was a wonderful young man we knew while he was in high school. At that time we knew him as *Mitch.* He was a good athlete and an excellent student who had become an outstanding physician at a world class cancer research hospital in Pennsylvania. We knew him and his family and had prayed for him when he developed and beat cancer while he was in college. *These two outstanding physicians spent hours talking with us on the telephone and gave us advice we would have been lost without. We owe both of them so much. How much is a life worth?*

On Friday, December 17, Jean and I had an appointment with the doctor who only three days earlier had indicate Jean had ovarian cancer. Dr. Knight discussed Jean's condition with us and told us the next step was surgery. She said she could perform the operation, but she recommended Dr. Goodman, a physician in Allentown, Pennsylvania. She had dealt with him on other cases and indicated the results were good. We agreed and while we waited she called his office and made an appointment for

December 27. As we left Dr. Knight's office, we began to feel there was a chance Jean would beat the cancer. Jean still had hope that the growths on her ovaries were not cancer. However, I felt that was unrealistic. There was just too much consistent evidence indicating ovarian cancer!

That afternoon Jean's good luck continued. We received a telephone call from Dr. Goodman's office indicating Jean's appointment had been changed to Monday, December 20…. seven days earlier than the original appointment. That evening we contacted the two physicians who were giving us advice. One of them evaluated Dr. Goodman's education, experience, and certifications—*one of only 600 physicians in the USA who is "board certified" in both oncology and gynecology!* He recommended Dr. Goodman highly and without reservations. The other physician who was advising us was also board certified in oncology and gynecology, and he knew Dr. Goodman personally and professionally. He also recommended Dr. Goodman highly. In addition, both physicians also had nothing but praise for— The Schuylkill Valley Hospital in Allentown, Pennsylvania—the hospital where Dr. Goodman did surgery.

We had two full days to rest and prepare ourselves for the Monday, December 20 appointment with Dr. Goodman. But how do you prepare for something like this? We tried to keep busy, so we occupied ourselves with the things we usually did on weekends—and I tried my best to comfort Jean. Many other people also tried to comfort her with cards, flowers, telephone calls, and visits. Some of them would also say to me: *"How are you doing?*" But not in the *"matter of fact"* way people normally greet each other. There was deep concern in their voices and I could see it on their faces.

That weekend Jean and I went to church, but not together. She went to a Roman Catholic mass, and I attended a Saturday evening Lutheran service. During the service I put a note in the collection basket requesting that the congregation pray for Jean. That was the best thing I did that weekend, and it produced results quickly. I received several wonderful telephone calls from the pastor expressing his concern and offering assistance if we needed it. Jean was included on the church's prayer list and remains on the list today, more than a year later. Many friends and family members told us they were praying for Jean, and they also put her name on the prayer lists of the churches they attended. *From the very beginning I believed and still believe these prayers from many people of different faiths helped Jean. Perhaps it was merely the knowledge that so many people cared about Jean, but I think it was more than good intentions from good people.*

When we realized that Jean probably had cancer, we immediately thought of my mother's experiences with lung cancer. My mother developed lung cancer in 1976 and died two years later on November 28, 1978—the day after our 13th wedding anniversary. Jean and I had vivid memories of the suffering my mother endured during those two years. Chemotherapy may have given my mother a few more months, perhaps even an entire year, but it is difficult to determine the true value of time secured by medical technology if the time is filled with pain and suffering.

Our situation was further complicated by an obvious issue that had to be faced. Christmas was only a few days off. In addition to all the other issues that needed attention, Jean was upset because Christmas would not be the happy event the entire family, especially grandchildren, looked forward to for so long. I remember Jean fixating on this and adding: *"What a terrible time to get sick."* In the midst of all the other issues we were dealing with, we had to decide *"what to do about Christmas."* For me this was a trivial matter that I was prepared to ignore, but I could not ignore any issue that added to Jean's emotional problems. So I came up with a solution—the rest of the family would celebrate Christmas on December 25, but Jean and I would, if necessary, celebrate Christmas two or three weeks later and call it *"Greek Christmas."* I reminded Jean that I was born and raised Greek Catholic, not Roman Catholic, and *"the Greeks"* celebrate Christmas two weeks after the Romans. I know there is some truth in this and remember at least acknowledging the later Greek Christmas as a child. Even if it was not completely true, it sounded good and it provided Jean with extra time to prepare for Christmas. I also told Jean that our grandchildren would love the idea because they would celebrate Christmas twice. Jean liked the idea so I presented it to our daughters Suzy and Lisa. They also supported the idea.

At least one problem was solved, or at least it was delayed for a few weeks. There were several other important things I did that weekend before our appointment with Dr. Goodman. Saturday and Sunday mornings I went to the fitness center to *"workout."* I spent two to three hours there both days and used the exercise bike, stretched, and did flexibility, strength and floor exercises. I went to church Saturday evening, something I started doing several years ago because it *"freed up"* Sunday mornings for time at the fitness center. I rely on exercise to clear my mind and reduce stress and depression. I also prepared a *to do list.* I started preparing *to do lists* while I was an undergraduate student because there was so much to do and too little time to do it! Jean was often irritated by my lists, especially after I retired. She would tell me *"retired people do not need to do lists."* Since we discovered Jean had cancer, I not only prepared many *to do lists,* I began preparing lists of questions and medications, files with Jean's medical records, and a detailed calendar.

The lists I prepared that weekend helped me focus my thinking and organize the many things I needed to do. Money was one of my chief concerns, resulting in a wide range of questions, especially about insurance coverage. I knew Jean's medical costs would total several hundred thousand dollars during the next year, and our medical and drug insurances would cover much of the cost, but I did not know how much. I also knew from personal experience that medical insurance companies have rules that seem to defy logic and can be very unforgiving if any are violated. Therefore, as soon as I realized it was likely Jean had cancer, I called my medical insurance company and described her symptoms and the surgery that was being considered. I spent more than an hour on the telephone and was greatly relieved by what I heard. I also learned something that surprised me. An outstanding hospital located in Pennsylvania within ninety miles of our home was not included in our insurance coverage!

I knew my insurance excluded some physicians, including some who were excellent, but I did not realize that an entire hospital could be excluded. Hearing this Jean became very angry, demanding to be taken to a hospital in New York City. We had not even decided on the physician we wanted, but she made up her mind that she would settle only for the best or rather what she thought was the best. I told her we knew nothing about the hospital she suggested, and it could be months before she would be seen by an appropriate physician. By that time she could be dead or her cancer could have advanced sufficiently for a cure to be impossible! I also pointed out that three physicians had recommended Dr. Goodman, and we had not even given him a chance to evaluate her condition and suggest a treatment strategy. Hearing this she became a bit more cooperative, but she insisted that we had terrible medical insurance.

My medical insurance continued after I retired from PENN STATE, and it covered both of us. I always believed that PENN STATE had an excellent fringe benefit package, especially the medical insurance. It was not surprising that Jean became angry and unreasonable. She was faced with a future that at best included major surgery and probably chemotherapy. *That was the best she could expect, but there was a distinct possibility she would simply die within the next few months. I know this was on her mind because we discussed the possibility this could be the last few months of her wonderful life.*

We did not sleep much Friday, Saturday, or Sunday evening. In fact, it was weeks before either of us had a restful sleep. The medications we were both taking to improve our emotional states and help us sleep provided little, if any, help! Without realizing it, we developed a *"new schedule"* or *"pattern of behavior"* that weekend that lasted several months. Every evening we watched several hours of mind numbing television followed by an eight to ten hour period in and out of bed—*hardly a restful sleep.* The next morning we would always have breakfast together. Preparation of breakfast became my responsibility as it is to this day. Breakfast conversation was the same every morning. We discussed how well we slept, how Jean felt, and what our plans were for the day.

Monday, December 20 arrived and at the assigned time, we found ourselves in Dr. Goodman's office. When he walked in, we were shocked by his appearance. He was tall, thin, smiling and very, very young. He reviewed Jean's medical record, especially the test results from the previous week, and indicated he was optimistic about her chances. He also said he did surgery on Thursdays and would like to schedule Jean for Thursday, December 23. He described the surgery in detail and indicated he would leave the appendix in. I questioned this and he said it was up to Jean. Jean asked his preference and he said he would rather not remove it. Jean agreed.

Dr. Goodman went on to say Jean would remain in the hospital for four or five days following surgery. He then began to discuss chemotherapy, which, at this point, seemed a certainty to me. If chemotherapy was needed, it should start approximately four weeks after surgery. There would be six treatments: one every three weeks, and each treatment would require three to four hours. I remember asking why chemotherapy could not start sooner before any remaining cancer cells had a chance to spread. He responded by saying Jean needed a month to recover from the surgery so she would have the strength needed to tolerate the chemotherapy. At no time did Dr. Goodman say it was certain Jean had cancer; but he did not leave much doubt, at least not in my mind.

Prior to leaving Dr. Goodman's office, a pre-admission testing and screening appointment was made for that afternoon, at the hospital where the surgery would be done. In addition, a follow up appointment was scheduled for 10 am on January 13, 2005. After leaving Dr. Goodman's office, we drove directly to the hospital for the testing and screening. The staff at the hospital was wonderful. *One nurse in admissions really lifted our spirits. She told us that Dr. Goodman was an excellent doctor and she added, "If you want to know who the good doctors are, ask a nurse." She also said, "Dr. Goodman looks like he is twelve years old" then, after a short pause, she added, "but I could marry him." At the time, Dr. Goodman was in his early forties, but he did look like a kid!*

We were still very anxious and upset, but we were delighted with the progress we made. I remember saying over and over again, *"things could not have gone any better."* We kept *"counting our blessings,"* which at this point meant reviewing all the good things that happened after receiving the initial devastating news. We were lucky Jean's *"condition"* was discovered early—*or so we thought.* Our friends and family helped us find a great doctor, and from the time of Jean's initial appointment *(December 14)* to the time of surgery *(December 23)* would be only nine days. *Based upon my limited knowledge of the medical system, that was a remarkably quick response time.*

After the testing and screening procedures were completed, Jean began calling people with the news ... family first, then friends. That evening we called the two doctors who had given us such helpful advice. We told them surgery was scheduled for December 23 and we thanked them. *We thanked them many times, we thanked our friends who put us in touch with them, and we thanked God.*

The next day I made up a very long *to do list* and immediately started working on the tasks I had just compiled. The first thing I did was telephone the companies that administered our medical and drug insurances to confirm we were operating within all the rules and guidelines that applied to Jean's situation. After that, I reserved a room at a motel near the hospital. We would arrive the day before surgery, so Jean would not be subjected to a one hour trip prior to surgery and we would not risk missing the surgery or arriving late because of bad road conditions. *(During December, highways can become hazardous very quickly in*

Pennsylvania. Even small, localized storms can make highways dangerous, resulting in accidents and traffic delays.)

The day before Jean's surgery, we called the hospital as required and confirmed the arrangements for the big day: no food or liquids from 10 pm the night before surgery and arrive at 5:30 am and report directly to the surgery admission/registration area. We arrived at the motel early so we could check in and still have time to go out for dinner. After the meal we returned to the motel and watched television for the rest of the evening. The next morning we woke up very early—actually we did not sleep much that night. We arrived at the hospital around 5 am. The hospital was open, lights were on everywhere and we saw very few people. We went to the surgical admissions/registration area and they were ready for Jean. *In a few minutes a nurse came for Jean; we hugged, kissed and told each other "I love you." I assured her that "everything will be fine" as she left.*

The hospital had a large waiting room for family and friends of patients undergoing surgery. I knew I would be there for several hours, so I found a comfortable location and sat down. One of the nurses told me Dr. Goodman would talk to me after the surgery was completed. In addition, the people working at the admissions desk said they could supply me with information regarding Jean's status: not medical information, just information about where she was in the surgery schedule. For example, when I asked, I was told the time surgery began. I don't remember the exact time, but I do recall *"timing"* the surgery.

Sally and her daughter Lori arrived shortly after the start of surgery. I told them Jean was in surgery and we sat down to wait. I had plenty of reading material and I also brought snacks and drinks. *When I determined the surgery had been in progress for two hours, I told Sally and Lori: "This is a good sign. If Dr. Goodman had cut Jean open and found an impossible situation, such as obvious cancer in many areas, he would have simply ended the procedure. If that had happened, it would have required less than two hours!" They agreed and we continued to wait.*

I have a difficult time remembering telephone numbers, addresses, names of people and birthdays; but I have no difficulty remembering all the details surrounding painful events. For example, Sally and I had a disagreement while sitting in the waiting room. Sally knew I planned on staying close to Jean from the time she entered the hospital until the time she left and returned home. This meant I would *"miss Christmas"* for the first time in my life. Jean, my two daughters and I agreed we would celebrate *"Greek Christmas"* two weeks after December 25th, the day when most Americans celebrate Christmas. Sally said it was reasonable to have a delayed Christmas, but I should not be by myself on Christmas Eve and Christmas Day. She went on to say I could at least come to her house for a meal on both days. I said "no," I wanted to be near my wife and my presence would be a distraction at any Christmas event I attended. I thought Sally felt guilty about celebrating Christmas while her sister was in the hospital recovering from major surgery.

After sitting in the waiting room for more than three hours, the receptionist told me Jean was out of surgery. She escorted Sally and me to a small room with a table and several chairs and said Dr. Goodman would be in to see us in a few minutes. In a short time Dr. Goodman arrived, shook my hand, and sat down. He was smiling as he sat down and told us the surgery went very well. He described what he found and said there were no surprises. *He was certain the mass on one ovary was cancer, but he was not sure about the mass on the other ovary. He cautioned us by saying everything he removed would be sent to a laboratory for analysis, and he would give Jean and me the results of the biopsy when we saw him for the follow up appointment on January 13. The meeting with Dr. Goodman lasted only a few minutes. When it was over we shook hands and I thanked him for all he had done for Jean. He smiled and left.*

I went back to the receptionist and asked when Jean would be out of recovery and in her own room. She said it would be several hours, and she suggested that I get something for lunch and go home for a few hours. I agreed and told them I was staying at a motel a short distance away. Sally and I began walking toward the hospital cafeteria. Her daughter Lori had already left. Before we arrived at the cafeteria, I went outside to call Suzy and Lisa and give them the latest news about their mother. I remember it was very cold outside. I am not certain why I went outside to make the calls—either cell phones were not allowed in that area of the hospital, or my cell phone would not work inside the hospital.

I called both daughters and gave them the information I had just received from Dr. Goodman. Lisa and Suzy were glad to hear the news, but they were both frightened. They were not surprised the doctor confirmed at least one mass was cancer. Suzy had an additional issue which we previously discussed. She was deeply concerned she might also develop ovarian cancer. She asked me if I had an opportunity to discuss this with Dr. Goodman. I told her I was focused on her mother and that issue would have to wait a few months.

After talking with Lisa and Suzy, Sally and I finally made it to the hospital cafeteria. I was happy to see the cafeteria had a nice selection of good food…. I knew I would be eating all of my meals there for several days.

After we ate, Sally left and I went back to the motel for a nap. I returned to the hospital around 3 or 4 pm and went directly to Jean's room. She was out of the recovery room and she was very drowsy. *I repeatedly told her the surgery was successful.* As time past she became more alert. She said I should go get something to eat. *(I miss very few meals, so I do not know why people are so concerned about me having enough to eat!)* I was happy to do that but I had more than food in mind.

I wanted to buy Jean one or two small Christmas presents that she could appreciate while she was in the hospital. The hospital had a nice gift shop, so I knew I could find something appropriate. I immediately saw a small ornamental tree which was about eighteen inches tall. It was perfect. The branches appeared to be covered in a series of clear crystal pieces. It would look beautiful in Jean's room—

it was not a Christmas decoration, but it could still be "our Christmas tree." There were many other wonderful items in the gift shop, but I especially liked the Willow Tree (registered trade name) display. Again, I found an ideal gift. It was a piece titled "Promise," which was simply a man and woman embracing, her right hand behind his neck and his left arm around her waist. More could be written about the "Promise," but words could never fully describe it or the significance it had for me.

I was excited about the presents as I rushed back to Jean's room without eating dinner. Jean loved both presents and cried when seeing them. She especially liked the "Promise." This was the first time I was able to make Jean happy since she received the awful news! We both cherish these two small Christmas presents and we always will. They are on display in our Pottsville home with many other beautiful pieces Jean and I have purchased over the years, but only Jean and I fully appreciate their special meaning.

The next day was December 24 and the hospital was deserted. The gift shop, the cafeteria, the halls and sitting areas were nearly empty. Jean and I were about to spend some quality time in her room, but we loved it when Suzy, Lisa, and our four grandchildren showed up to pay her a visit.

Occasionally I would leave Jean's room and walk around the hospital. Jean was healing and she needed to sleep. As evening approached I was extremely depressed. I was with Jean—exactly where I wanted to be—but the joy of Christmas was not in my heart. As I walked around I realized something surprising. This would be the first time in my life I would not attend a church service on Christmas. I thought about this for a while recalling my mother's religious beliefs and practices; I knew she had taken me to Christmas mass even when I was an infant! I based this not only on what I knew of my mother, but also her family. I recalled that her mother, my maternal grandmother, went to mass every day and even died in church during mass. This made me even more unhappy because I would not leave the hospital while Jean was there, not even to attend a Christmas service. Suddenly I realized every hospital has a chapel—at least I could pray in the chapel on Christmas Eve.

I easily found the chapel, but when I opened the door and walked in I was shocked at what I saw. A priest was standing directly in front of me less than thirty feet away, and a Roman Catholic mass was about to begin. But this was not a Christmas mass. There were large pictures of a young man on display and people sitting in the church were certainly not celebrating. They were all sad and many were crying. Seeing my hesitation, the priest gestured for me to come in, sit, and attend the mass that was about to begin. I knew this was not a mass for the general public. Initially I assumed this mass was to mourn the passing of the young man whose picture was so prominently displayed. As the mass continued I learned the young man was a burn victim who was being treated in the hospital. But there were more surprises. He had been covered with a flammable fluid and set on fire by an unknown person or persons! I was also shocked to discover he had attended a high school in Pottsville, Pennsylvania just a few miles from our home.

During the mass the priest gave everyone a chance to speak. There were many tears and there was anger. The males who spoke were especially angry. I could understand this because I was also angry. A little later, the priest asked everyone to extend a greeting to those around them—a common practice during a Christian mass or religious service. This took much longer than it would in a typical mass because these people "were family" gathered to pray for a loved one who was near death. Family members even approached me with hand extended and thanked me for coming. I apologized for intruding on their special mass, but every one of them indicated they were happy I was there. For a short time I forgot about Jean and prayed for a young man I had never met. I still remember him in my prayers.

After mass I went to the cafeteria for my Christmas Eve meal. Surprisingly I felt better, but I didn't know why. I sat and was about to eat my meal when several people who were at the mass sat near me and we began talking. We were the only people in a rather large eating area. I introduced myself and told them about Jean's surgery and her condition. And then they told me about the young man they all loved. They described what they knew about how he was intentionally set on fire. They also said he was in a coma. I believe his coma was induced so that his mind was protected from the extreme pain his body was experiencing. One family member gave me two numbers that I cannot confirm, but I still remember. The burns covered 90% of the young man's body and he had only a 10% chance of survival. The engineer in me made it easy to remember: 90% plus 10% equals 100% in the terrible calculus of this young man's life. I reacted very quickly to these numbers because I could not accept them! I told them I could remember when I was a tough young man about the age of their family member and "I don't give a damn what the doctors say. I know that the 10% number is wrong. He is going to live!" I remember this so clearly because I was angry and I clenched both hands into "tight fists," which I only do when I am angry. Never have I been so angry, but I have no idea why I was angry or who I was angry with.

I left the cafeteria and told Jean what had occurred—an unexpected mass in the chapel, a burn victim from our home town currently in the hospital, the manner in which he was burned and his condition. She responded by saying that "God wanted you there." Jean frequently sees "God at work" in many small or trivial events, but this was such an amazing event that even other family members arrived at the same conclusion. I doubt God played a role in my arriving at the chapel on Christmas Eve when I did—or my becoming involved with a family looking for hope while I was on a separate quest for hope—but I can not dismiss the possibility. To this day, this event gives me hope, hope there is a God and hope that Jean will beat the cancer she is fighting. And my hope has been amplified by what has happened since that Christmas Eve mass.

Anyone with writing experience knows I should wait until the proper point in the chronology to describe what became of this young man. But the news is so good, I just can not wait. The writer must defer to how I feel. The young man survived and today is a student at an institution of higher learning! I am an optimistic person. I know there is always hope, even when all hope seems to have *vanished! This young man's survival proves it! I hope this young man lives a long, productive life. But I doubt he will ever appreciate how on Christmas Eve 2004, his tragedy intersected with the tragedy my family was experiencing, and it gave us hope when we needed it the most. Perhaps Jean was right when she said, "God wanted you there."*

The next few days were uneventful—*even Christmas Day*. On December 27, 2004 Jean was discharged and we returned to our home in Pottsville. We were both happy to be home enjoying family—especially our grandchildren. The surgery was in the past and Jean needed to regain her strength so she could face the ordeal of chemotherapy that would begin in a few weeks. New Year's Eve was approaching but it didn't really matter. We had stopped partying on the eve of the New Year a long time ago. *Usually we celebrated the arrival of the New Year with a fine meal and an end of the year toast. This year we had a simple meal, but we did have a toast. I do not remember the exact words, but I remember the sentiment. Thank God 2004 is over, and hopefully 2005 will be a good year—a happy year. <u>We never expected a year like 2004 and we will never forget it!</u>*

CHAPTER 5

Chemotherapy #1 and #2
January to February 2005

Dr. Goodman said Jean would need four weeks to recover from surgery before she would be strong enough for her first chemotherapy treatment (*chemo #1*). I had hoped the chemotherapy could start sooner, believing that any delay would give remaining cancer cells a chance to spread. I was beginning to learn, however, that Dr. Goodman's advice was sound. At the beginning of January it was clear Jean needed time to recover physically and emotionally. Besides, the entire family wanted Jean to be ready for Christmas: the *"Greek Christmas"* we decided to celebrate prior to Jean's surgery.

Two weeks after the traditional Christmas most Americans celebrate, our family gathered at Suzy and John's house to celebrate our Christmas. I really don't know the exact date when Greek Christmas is celebrated, but it is later than December 25. Even the term Greek Christmas is not appropriate, although it is widely used and recognized in many areas of Pennsylvania. There were ten of us gathered around the large dining room table—Suzy's family, Lisa's family, Jean, and myself. I made sure that Daniel was next to me as we prepared to say grace. I wanted to say something special, thanking God for helping Jean and all of us through a difficult time. I immediately started crying; and Daniel who understood that his grandmother was in danger of losing her life, followed my example. Our celebration was not the joyous event I had hoped for. How could it be, knowing this could be Jean's last Christmas with the family?

We all knew Jean might not survive, especially when we learned more about ovarian cancer. Jean and I immersed ourselves in reading about this disease and what we read did not give us much hope. I was especially concerned when I read that ovarian cancer is often referred to as "the silent killer." Jean's only symptoms were bloating and abdominal pressure, and she saw a physician a short time after that. Adding to our frustration was the knowledge that Jean had annual PAP tests and mammograms as well as a colonoscopy, an endoscopy, a CAT scan and several blood tests in the eight months prior to the diagnosis of ovarian cancer. Also, during that period she was examined by a gynecologist and a gastroenterologist. How could two doctors and many medical tests fail to detect the cancer sooner? Or does ovarian cancer spread so quickly that in a period of just a few months it reached both ovaries? I also wondered if it had spread to other locations in her body. There were answers to these questions and others that raced through our minds, but honest answers would have done nothing except increase our anxiety to even higher levels.

Jean was thinking of her death, and we discussed that possibility as we reflected on the value of our lives. It was painful to balance the accomplishments of a good life against the possibility of an early death, and yet it was useful to consider and plan for the end. Jean is rarely concerned about financial issues. She leaves that to me and spends money freely. That's why I was surprised in early January when she told me she would sign up for Social Security benefits as soon as she became eligible. Jean said she did not know how long she would live so it made "good sense" to apply for benefits at the earliest possible date. I knew exactly what she meant and I agreed with her. Previously we agreed to wait until age sixty-five before either of us would apply for Social Security benefits—and suddenly she was announcing her intention to apply for benefits three years earlier, when she turned sixty-two! She went on to say the additional money should be used to pay off our condo in South Carolina. It seemed to me she was concerned about my finances if she died.

On January 13, 2005 Jean had her post surgery appointment with Dr. Goodman. This was a multi-purpose examination: evaluate healing after surgery, discuss biopsy report, take blood samples for testing, and set up the schedule for chemotherapy, if it was needed. Jean went into the examination room while I sat in the waiting room. As soon as her examination was over, a nurse asked me to go back with my wife. *I could see from the expression on the nurse's face that the news was not good. Jean was crying when I arrived. She had already learned that the biopsy revealed her cancer was Stage III B.*

This meant Jean's cancer was advanced.

Dr. Goodman patiently described the biopsy results:

- Serious carcinoma on both ovaries
- Serious carcinoma on uterus
- Seventeen lymph nodes tested (all free of malignancy)
- Serious carcinoma on the omentum (a 0.7 cm nodule)

The results were devastating. We had hoped for a Stage II result, but the cancer was far more advanced, resulting in a Stage III classification. The only good news was that the cancer had not spread to the lymph nodes. Cancer can spread through the blood system and through the lymph node system. The fact that seventeen lymph nodes were free of cancer meant that it had not "jumped" the barrier separating the two systems. After Dr. Goodman described the biopsy results, we began to ask questions. Jean asked how likely it was that she would be cured. Dr. Goodman said "about 40%." This led to a discussion of life expectancy. Dr. Goodman said the average life expectancy for someone with advanced ovarian cancer is about five years. I asked what the standard deviation was. He said it was a good question but that he did not know. Standard deviation is a measure of variability and I hoped it would be very large. If it was large, Jean would at least have some chance for a long life. There was one last significant statistic presented by Dr. Goodman in response to a question from Jean: "What if I decide not to take chemotherapy?" Still smiling, Dr. Goodman said, "That's a very a good question. You will die in about one year." I stopped breathing as I waited for Jean to speak. She said, "OK I'll take the chemotherapy." Dr. Goodman had handled it exactly the right way. Rather than telling Jean to take the chemotherapy, he gave her the hard facts and waited for her to make the decision.

There was one last issue to consider. Did Jean want a port surgically placed under her skin between a shoulder and breast? A port is essentially a two way valve which is connected to an appropriate artery allowing easy insertion of a needle when extracting blood for testing or when placing fluids into the blood supply—as required for chemotherapy. Jean liked the idea of having a port because there had been so many times when a physician or nurse had a difficult time *"finding a vein"* during a medical procedure. Surgery for installation of the port was scheduled for January 25, two days before her first chemotherapy treatment.

Installation of the port was done on an outpatient basis and required less than one hour. I was sitting in the waiting room— the same waiting room I sat in on December 23 when Jean had major surgery—when a nurse called my name and directed me to a small room. She told me the doctor would join me in a few minutes. Dr. Goodman entered the room and told me everything was fine and Jean would be ready to go home in two or three hours.

This was his last surgery of a very long day and he was clearly exhausted. I thanked him for all he had done for Jean. Then I told him, "I could never do what you do … to make life and death decisions on a daily basis, telling people about their chances of living and dying … and to tell a family that a loved one died … I simply could not do it." This was the first time Dr. Goodman spoke to me while holding back tears. He said "There are times when I do everything right and the patient still dies. I just get so angry."

Doctors and nurses are the ultimate caregivers, and they share the emotions of the patient and the patient's family. They have chosen a profession that requires them to behave according to a set of norms that I could not live with. They must remain calm and stay detached in the face of gut-wrenching experiences. It takes more than exceptional intellectual ability to be a physician like Dr. Goodman. It takes compassion, confidence, and an inner strength that few people have. *Jean and I thank God for many things and from December 2004 to this day, we thanked God for Dr. Goodman and the wonderful staff that assists him.*

On January 27, 2005, Jean and I once again arrived at the medical suite Dr. Goodman and his staff use in Allentown, Pennsylvania. But this time we had a new set of anxieties. This was the day of Jean's first chemotherapy treatment. In a short time we were directed to the room where the chemotherapy was to be administered. Nancy, a delightful young nurse with special training related to the care of cancer patients, greeted us and with great deliberation began to set up for the therapy. I was encouraged to stay with Jean for the entire procedure. Although we were apprehensive about what was to follow, Nancy made us feel at ease. She was always pleasant, informative and she laughed when I told her she is known as *"The Chemo Queen."* Preparing the equipment used for administration of the two chemotherapy drugs that Jean would receive required only a few minutes.

We learned much that day. For example, other medicines could be included with the cancer fighting drugs being fed into Jean's body intravenously. These supplements to the chemotherapy drugs were adjusted according to how Jean felt—what she was experiencing—as well as the side effects she experienced since the last chemotherapy treatment. *We also learned something else that day. Blood samples had been taken during the January 13 appointment with Dr. Goodman and the results were given to us. Jean's CA125 had dropped from 1,006 prior to surgery to 116! Cancer cells could still be present, but the surgery worked! For the first time since Jean received a diagnosis of cancer, we had reason to hope and to celebrate.* Even as we enjoyed the moment, I pondered the uncertainty of medical tests. There are so many false positives and false negatives associated with medical testing. Could our good news simply be a mistake (*a bad data point*)? By this time I had read hundreds of pages about ovarian cancer and the methods used to "*detect*" and "*measure*" it. I could not imagine how this reading could be false, but I could not be certain it was correct until at least one more blood test confirmed the results.

The first chemotherapy took four hours and Jean was tired when it was over. There was also anxiety because we did not know what side effects she would encounter. Dr. Goodman, Nancy "*The Chemo Queen,*" and other medical professionals in the medical suite assured us there are usually mild side effects after the first and second chemotherapy treatments. At the same time however, Dr. Goodman told us not to travel to South

Carolina until after the second chemotherapy treatment—Just in case something happens. *"Just in case" is one of the wild cards of life that can not be fully understood or explained, and only a fool ignores.*

While driving home we stopped in Fogelsville for our celebration. We went to a nice restaurant for a late lunch. This may not sound like much of a celebration, but it was wonderful. We toasted Dr. Goodman and his staff, we toasted the good news, and we toasted each other. Sounds a bit *"corny,"* especially since we toasted with glasses of water and diet soda. We also enjoyed ourselves for the first time in six weeks. The restaurant is part of a national chain of unique restaurants with a great menu including *"breakfast throughout the day."* Jean loves this and frequently orders from the breakfast menu, even late in the afternoon. When entering any of these restaurants, you first pass through a large gift shop area with a wide range of items—candy, bread, CDs, clothing, reading material, toys and much, much more! Jean always shops in the gift shop, and it is rare for her to not buy something.

This was a "Perfect Storm" kind of day for shopping and I remember Jean's logic for filling several large bags with a wide assortment of items, especially "stuff for the grandkids!"

1. *We did not have much of a Christmas.*

2. *We did not buy many Christmas presents for our grandchildren.*

3. *The prices were excellent—prices were lowered to get rid of Christmas inventory.*

4. *She had not spent much money in the last six weeks.*

The real reason for the shopping spree was Jean had received good news that meant she might survive—perhaps even be cured of ovarian cancer. I was so swept up in the moment that I bought a large cowboy hat. It was a great price and I liked the cowboy look because Jean said it makes me look sexy. After leaving the restaurant and gift shop, we traveled about an hour before arriving at our home in Pottsville. Of course, Jean was on the cell phone the entire time with family members and friends describing the chemotherapy experience and giving them the good news regarding the CA125 results. Once we got home, Jean settled in for a relaxing evening. By the end of the evening, she began to experience some side effects. Her cheeks were red and her stomach was slightly upset. Also, she did not sleep well that night. Was it anxiety or a side effect of the chemotherapy?

The side effects lasted only three or four days and as Dr. Goodman and his staff predicted, they were not severe. Of course, this was only the first treatment and five more were planned. Jean and I knew the side effects of chemotherapy were cumulative: they become progressively worse after each treatment. So once she felt better, we started doing things that we enjoy: eating out, spending quality time with our grandchildren, and planning our next trip to South Carolina.

Approximately one week after the chemotherapy treatment we returned to Dr. Goodman's medical suite in Allentown so that blood samples could be taken for additional testing. During each *"chemotherapy cycle"* two blood samples were drawn and analyzed; the first approximately three days prior to the day chemotherapy drugs were administered and the second approximately one week after. The first blood test includes CA125 results and the second test does not. More importantly, results of the first test are used as a *"stop-go"* signal for the next chemotherapy treatment. If the results suggest the patient has not sufficiently recovered from the previous chemotherapy treatment, the next treatment is delayed.

It was not necessary for us to return to Dr. Goodman's medical suite for the second blood test, but we frequently did. Blood testing laboratories are available in many places, but we wanted Dr. Goodman and his staff involved as deeply as possible in every aspect of Jean's battle against cancer. And so we made sure they had the opportunity to review and pass judgment on everything that could possibly have a relationship to Jean's cancer. We even informed them of food supplements Jean was considering. It may seem we were being too careful or just plain wasting our time, but I believe we did the right thing. I am also certain we will continue to ask Dr. Goodman to review all future medical conditions and medical procedures that could have any relationship to Jean's condition.

Jean and I had expected to travel to South Carolina between the first and second chemotherapy treatments and stay for a week to ten days, but Dr. Goodman told us we should remain in Pennsylvania, *"just in case something happens."* We enjoyed life between the first and second chemotherapy treatments, and the time passed quickly ... *but oh how I wanted to be in South Carolina!*

We knew Jean's chemotherapy treatments would become the *"center of our existence"* for months to come as we approached the second treatment. Of course there were minor variations, but the second treatment and all later treatments followed the same basic routine:

- *The pre-chemotherapy pelvic and rectal examination and discussions with Dr. Goodman or members of his staff came first. Blood samples were taken for testing and Jean's weight was recorded. This was something Jean approached with great concern, because she was gaining weight. This entire appointment lasted around two hours.*

- *Pre-chemotherapy medications (steroids) were taken the night before and morning of the treatment.*

- *Jean received her treatment three days after the pre-chemotherapy visit. After the first treatment, we were not at all apprehensive about the treatment itself—only the side effects which followed. Besides, "The Chemo Queen" made the three to four hour treatment as pleasant as possible. I sat near Jean during the appointment, although I would occasionally leave for a short walk or to shop at a nearby drug* store. One other detail should be mentioned: Jean usually brought a snack for Dr. Goodman and his staff.

- Approximately seven days after the chemotherapy treatment, blood was taken for the second test. One other point should be made about our frequent trips to the Allentown region to satisfy Jean's medical needs. We went to our favorite restaurant in Fogelsville after most of Jean's appointments. We enjoyed the food and Jean loved shopping in the gift shop after we ate.

Chemotherapy #2 was administered on February 16, 2005 and it was uneventful. We were much less apprehensive than we were prior to and during chemotherapy #1. Jean was doing well, so Dr. Goodman said we could travel to South Carolina after the second treatment. In fact, he encouraged us to go and have a good time. *I remember this was the first time he made comments about "the quality of life." I know exactly what that phrase means, but I was not sure why he now raised the issue and even stressed its importance.* I was afraid to pursue this with him because Jean became irritable with me when I asked questions, especially questions that could strike her as being inappropriate or, God forbid, might imply that I was questioning Dr. Goodman's judgment! *But why was Dr. Goodman telling us "Quality of Life" was important? Did he believe a happy person had a better chance of surviving cancer, or did he think Jean's chances were so bleak we might as well enjoy the time she had left?*

Our vehicle was packed for our trip to South Carolina, so when the second chemotherapy treatment was completed, we said our good-byes and headed south. I knew Jean would be tired, so we only drove 250 miles the first day and spent the evening in Fredericksburg, Virginia. Jean was beginning to experience side effects, but they were mild as Dr. Goodman and his staff had predicted. We had a meal at a restaurant and returned to our motel room for the evening. The next day Jean's face and abdomen were again red and she experienced fatigue and nausea, but we had no difficulty completing our trip. We arrived at our condo mid-afternoon that day.

Our condo has three bedrooms and a fantastic view of the ocean. It is located in Ocean Creek—a residential community on the northern edge of Myrtle Beach, South Carolina. We always receive an emotional lift when we arrive because we both love South Carolina, the ocean and "our beach." This time our arrival had special meaning because it was the first time we were able to return to South Carolina since we learned Jean had ovarian cancer.

The next day we called Dr. Goodman's office for the latest CA125 results. CA125 results were frequently the last piece of information to be transmitted from the laboratory to Dr. Goodman's office, but the results had arrived. Jean's CA125 was 1,006 prior to surgery and 116 prior to chemotherapy #1. But the latest result, based upon a blood sample prior to the second treatment, was 30! *It was now certain that Jean's condition was improving.*

The week following chemotherapy #2, Jean experienced a wide range of side effects: flushed face and abdomen, trouble sleeping, puffy eyes, queasy feeling in the stomach and constipation. *In spite of all of this, on the second day after chemotherapy, Jean said, "Thank you God," because things were not as bad as she expected.* Early in March we returned to Pennsylvania and began to prepare for the next treatment.

The previous two months were very stressful for Jean and me and there was one constant missing from our lives. My father was in Florida with Rosie and Pete, so we did not have the opportunity to visit him at the Laurels. Of course we called him frequently, especially after the side effects of chemotherapy left Jean's body.

CHAPTER 6

Chemotherapy #3, #4, #5 and #6
March 1 to July 18, 2005

The next four treatments followed the same routine used during the first two treatments. But the side effects were now far worse— far more intense than anything Jean experienced earlier—and she was experiencing several new side effects that were horrible. Also, her appearance was changing and this only added to her emotional pain.

Jean's third chemotherapy treatment took place on March 10, 2005. Her hair was beginning to fall out, but that was easy to deal with … *at least I thought so.* Jean bought two wigs and ordered several head coverings and hats. A few weeks later she had her hair cut very short by a good friend who for many years was also her hair dresser. For them, it was a sad experience. The hair dresser cried as she cut the little hair that Jean had left. In all honesty, changes in Jean's appearance did not bother me in the least. I still loved her and she was still beautiful. It may seem strange but I was actually happy to see Jean's hair fall out. However, I never told her how I felt—it would have upset her deeply, perhaps even angered her! The chemicals used in chemotherapy kill fast growing cells in the body, including cancer cells. But chemotherapy is not perfect; it cannot be perfect, so it also kills other cells. The most obvious are cells related to maintaining and growing hair—and not just the hair on a person's head. *So right or wrong, I was happy to see Jean's hair fall out because it meant the chemotherapy was doing what it was designed to do—kill fast growing cells.*

As mentioned earlier, Jean was also gaining weight, but that must be placed into its proper context. Even at her highest weight, Jean was less overweight than most women we know who are approximately her age. Secondly, it was clear that Jean was far less active than she had been and this will certainly add pounds to anyone. The third reason Jean gained weight has some humor associated with it. We ate more and more frequently, and we ate more of the foods we loved but should not eat—cakes, cookies, snacks, and oh so much ice cream! A major food store near our home in Pennsylvania occasionally sells a high quality ice cream at a significant discount—*Buy One get One Free!* So one week I bought six half-gallons of ice cream—flavors we both loved. In just nine days we consumed the entire six half-gallons of ice cream. Obviously Jean was not the only one who had difficulty maintaining body weight while she was receiving chemotherapy.

Prior to her third chemotherapy treatment *Jean also began to complain about "chemo brain."* I read about this side effect of chemotherapy, but I did not take it seriously. In fact, I initially thought it was a joke—perhaps one only cancer survivors could appreciate. After more reading and listening to Jean discuss her symptoms with Dr. Goodman and his staff, I realized that *chemo brain* was real. It could be a significant condition and it may even be permanent. I find it difficult to describe *chemo brain* because it can surface in different ways resulting in a wide range of symptoms. A simple way to describe it is to state the obvious— *Chemo brain is any impairment in mental ability resulting from chemotherapy.* In some cases, cancer survivors who receive chemotherapy do not experience any *chemo brain* side effects; in other cases it can be extreme even disabling.

In March 2005 I could see only a few, very subtle signs of chemo brain in Jean. Of course my view may have been distorted by the other side effects she was experiencing after her third chemotherapy treatment. I could see her hair loss, but as far as I was concerned that was a minor inconvenience. *But the pain and discomfort she was experiencing exploded after her third treatment, and I could see the pain in her eyes and on her face.* Emotionally I could feel her pain and I wished there was some way for me to experience her physical pain, but that was one thing she could not share with me. Her constipation, nausea, difficulty sleeping were also far worse, making it even harder for her to endure pain. Not only were the side effects more severe; after each successive chemotherapy treatment they lasted longer, and after the third treatment they included *chemo brain.*

From everything I read and from what I was about to witness, chemo brain did not diminish a week or ten days after the chemotherapy treatment the way the other side effects did. Chemo brain had and continues to have a troubling permanence about it more than a year after it first occurred and more than four months since the last chemotherapy treatment. The specific *chemo brain* symptoms Jean experienced were as follows:

- *Inability to retrieve words, at times very simple words.*
- *Difficulty remembering the names of friends.*
- *Inability to focus for long periods of time, especially on complex issues.*
- *Forgetfulness—at times extreme short term memory problems.*

After the third chemotherapy treatment we received wonderful news. Jean's CA125 had fallen for the third time to a value of 13! This was phenomenal news because 35 or lower is considered normal. *Jean once again greeted good news by saying, "Thank you God."*

In April, prior to Jean's fourth treatment, Dr. Goodman indicated the latest research showed an additional round of chemotherapy *(beyond the six treatments originally planned)* could produce a significant improvement in the time duration cancer survivors remain *"cancer free."* He was careful to say the research had not yet matured sufficiently to confirm improvements in *"cure rates"* and *"average life expectancy values,"* but these seemed to be likely outcomes. *The additional round of chemotherapy that he recommended for Jean would consist of six to twelve treatments spaced one month apart and would be referred to as a "consolidation round."*

In spite of the severity of her side effects, March 2005 was a wonderful month. Jean's CA125 had fallen to normal levels for the first time and medical research had produced another weapon Jean could use in her battle against cancer: additional chemotherapy which Jean bravely agreed to. And there was one last enormous piece of good news we received in March:

Jean was officially in remission!

This meant Jean was free of all cancer symptoms—not yet cured, perhaps never cured; but you cannot move from *ADVANCED CANCER,* which she had only three months earlier, to *TOTALLY CURED* in one enormous step. *It simply cannot be done.* There are several steps and Jean had just taken a very big one. Three months earlier we were considering the real possibility that her life could end in months or perhaps in one or two years. Now we were seeing the benefits of all our efforts and all the pain she had endured. *We were now thinking, praying and hoping for a TOTAL CURE!*

But perhaps we were too optimistic. At least it seemed that way when Dr. Goodman responded to my following question: *"Does this mean Jean's chances for a total cure have increased from your initial estimate of 40%; and her average life expectancy was now more than five years?"* With a smile he said *"no."*

How could he possibly say "no" when we had received such good news and even Dr. Goodman said, *"Jean is responding well to chemotherapy"* and *"Jean is tolerating chemotherapy very well?"*

How could this brilliant, compassionate man of medicine shatter our newly found enthusiasm when my logic and newly developed understanding of cancer told me her chances were improving dramatically? I cannot and do not pretend to understand cancer, especially ovarian cancer, nearly as well as Dr. Goodman. However, I think he was intentionally lowering our expectations because it is better to be surprised by pleasant outcomes than to be crushed by unexpected bad news. I also believe that Dr. Goodman, like most doctors, was playing *"cover your ass."* I understand this, and if I was in his situation, I would do exactly the same thing. Medical professionals, especially physicians, must constantly guard themselves against legal action. And so, my opinion, which I shared with Jean, was and remains that Dr. Goodman has a natural tendency to error on the downside—*to overstate the negative and understate the positive.* I see the same behavior in so many instances, not just with Jean, but the medical experiences of my daughters, their children and in my own experiences with the medical community.

Jean had her fourth chemotherapy treatment on March 31 and her fifth on April 21. The pain and the side effects Jean experienced after her third chemotherapy treatment were terrible. But what she experienced after her fourth and fifth treatments was unbelievable, absolutely unbelievable. It broke my heart watching her suffer, and I couldn't do anything to help her—not a damn thing! Sure I could take care of the house, drive her to medical appointments and do many other things to make her life easier, but I could not ease her pain.

After the fourth treatment, Jean was so weak she could no longer write in her journal. Once she stopped keeping her journal, she never restarted. After other treatments we at least considered traveling to South Carolina, but not after the fourth treatment. She was too weak to travel, she was sick, and she had severe pain.

But even in times of darkness there can be light. Jean's CA125 continued to improve—it was 10 after the fourth treatment and 6 after her fifth treatment! It was this kind of good news that kept Jean going and which lifted both of our spirits.

For the entire month of April, Jean had pain in her legs—where it was the worst—but she also had terrible pain in her feet and her back. There were many times I would massage the areas where she was experiencing pain. Occasionally it helped, but other times it had little or no effect. Her pain always intensified in the evening—*the worst possible time*—right before she went to bed for the evening. She was having trouble sleeping and the medicines she took to help her sleep (*there were three*) did not provide much help. She also had medications for pain—over the counter products which Dr. Goodman approved. They provided only marginal relief.

The massages I gave Jean helped slightly and the addition of pain creams or lotions—*all over the counter products*—increased their effectiveness. Massages given by a therapist were far better than anything I could possibly do and there were other advantages. *Hilda, the woman Jean went to for massages, is a good friend, a free spirit and one of only three people Jean and I refer to* as "Saints." *Of course she is not a real saint, just a good friend with a good soul.*

Not only was Jean experiencing pain and other side effects, the chemotherapy drugs were also causing several problems with her blood. On April 22, the day after her fifth chemotherapy treatment, Jean received her first injection of a medicine designed to solve one of the problems. Chemotherapy had reduced her white blood count below acceptable limits and the injected medicine countered this by encouraging the production of white blood cells. *These shots were always given the day after chemotherapy.*

Jean also had a low red blood cell count that was treated with a second injected medicine. These injections were given weekly. *Dr. Goodman and his staff decided that I should give these injections. But I had never given an injection … and the thought of giving one scared the hell out of me! And so, I was given oral and written instructions on how to give the injections, but I insisted on more training.* I wanted to see a nurse give one of the injections. On April 28 we traveled to Dr. Goodman's office where Jean received the first of these injections, while I watched and took notes. I gave Jean the next four injections, *but I was always uneasy about doing it.* After that Jean's red blood cell count remained at acceptable levels.

Jean also had a third blood problem. Her liver enzymes were too high, but not dangerously high. This was a concern and was watched until they returned to normal in approximately six weeks. This was achieved without the benefit of any medicine or medical procedure.

Jean's sixty-second birthday was on April 24th, three days after her fifth treatment. I gave her two birthday cards—I always gave her more than one card—and a gift certificate for several massages. For the second year in a row, Jean was physically ill on her birthday. But this year we had hope. Perhaps next year we would have joy.

In March we had asked Dr. Goodman if we could deviate from the normal three week recovery period between chemotherapy treatments five and six. From the very beginning he said it would be all right. In fact he said it was a good idea— *once again stressing "Quality of Life."*

Jean needed about three weeks to recover sufficiently from the fifth chemotherapy treatment, and then she was able to travel to South Carolina. We spent the last two weeks of May there with our daughter Suzy and her family. We had a great time and Jean was beginning to regain her strength. I was greatly encouraged when she was able to walk several miles on the beach.

We returned home in plenty of time for Jean to complete the last treatment of the original six treatment chemotherapy round. The additional time we waited before the sixth treatment had allowed Jean's body time to recover. She still had pain and other side effects, but her energy level was much higher and she was sleeping better. *The sixth treatment was uneventful except for one thing: We had a pizza party at Dr. Goodman's office.* Several months earlier, I told his staff we would have a party to mark the day of what we thought would be Jean's last treatment. The party was enjoyable. It lifted our spirits and it marked the end of the first six treatments. *After a short pause, Jean would begin the consolidation round of treatments—six more chemotherapy treatments spaced one month apart rather than three weeks apart.*

It should be noted that Jean recovered from the sixth treatment quickly, and with less pain and fewer side effects than she experienced after the fourth and fifth treatments. The time we took for a vacation in South Carolina had extended the time between treatments five and six and this prevented a repeat of the agony she experienced earlier.

Pause, Evaluate and Plan

On June 6 Jean began to receive physical therapy designed for cancer survivors. She enjoyed the experience, but only went three times. She saw little benefit from the one-hour sessions.

On June 9 Jean had a major appointment with Dr. Goodman. Blood samples were drawn and she received a complete gynecological physical examination. A CAT scan was scheduled and we discussed the next round of chemotherapy—the consolidation round. *We were assured the side effects would be less severe for the consolidation round of chemotherapy treatments than they were for the original round. The following reasons were given:*

- *Jean would receive only one chemotherapy drug with each treatment rather than two drugs per treatment, as was the case with the original round.*

- *The treatments would be every four weeks instead of every three weeks.*

- *Jean was far healthier at the start of the consolidation round than she was at the start of the original round.*

- *Experience gained during the original round would help prevent side effects during the consolidation round.*

Aside from a longer interval between treatments, the routine for the consolidation treatments would be the same as it was for the original round of treatments:

- *Gynecological examination and blood drawn for testing— three days prior to the chemotherapy treatment.*

- *Pre-chemotherapy medications (steroids) the night before and morning of treatment.*

- *Chemotherapy treatment for three or four hours.*

- *Endure side effects and recover.*

- *Blood work approximately one week after chemotherapy.*

- *Continue to recover and wait for the next chemotherapy treatment.*

On July 13, the CAT scan was performed and we received the results from Dr. Goodman on July 18. Once again the news was good. *The CAT scan did not detect any problems, and Jean's latest CA125 was 6. <u>Jean was clearly in remission and we prayed it would continue.</u>*

CHAPTER 7

Six More Chemotherapy Treatments
July 19 to December 31, 2005

Jean approached the consolidation round of chemotherapy in good spirits and with little fear. Dr. Goodman was clearly a brilliant physician; everything he and his staff did and said was correct, and there was evidence—*good solid evidence*—that Jean was winning her battle with cancer.

It is difficult to think, write or speak of cancer without using the logic and language of warfare. I have frequently heard or read statements similar to one or more of the following:

- *A brave soul lost her battle with cancer.*
- *Another treatment was found in the war against cancer.*
- *A research center has uncovered additional information about the behavior of cancer cells that opens a new front in the war against cancer.*

There is a famous quotation about warfare which I believe applies to cancer:

There are no atheists in foxholes.

Similarly, there are no atheists in the war on cancer: the medical professionals, caregivers, family of survivors, and the survivors themselves. Jean and I have met more than one hundred of them since she developed cancer and every one of them, <u>every single one of them believes in God</u>. Cancer is such a formidable enemy, that it is difficult, perhaps even impossible, to confront it on a daily basis, without God or a Greater Presence providing strength, courage and comfort.

And so Jean and I prepared for the next round of chemotherapy and hoped it would be the last. Dr. Goodman and his staff were on our side, and this gave us great confidence. We knew they had enormous ability, and we knew they had great strength that came to them from the same source ours was derived from: *God.*

Jean received the first chemotherapy treatment of the consolidation round on July 28, 2005. Her second treatment took place at the end of August and shortly afterward we received another positive result: Jean's CA125 was still 6. She would receive four more treatments after that, always during the last week of the month.

In September our daughter Suzy and her family once again joined us in South Carolina. We returned from South Carolina at the end of September and Jean received her third treatment of the consolidation round. A few days later we received her latest blood test results. Her CA125 rose to 8 from a value of 6 the previous month. I was deeply concerned about this increase in the ovarian cancer marker, but I did not express this to Jean. She was doing so well, but I knew she was very fragile emotionally. I privately expressed my concerns to Dr. Goodman and his staff, and they told me not to worry. They told me *"any value below 20 is great."* They used words like *"glitch"* and *"anomaly"* to explain why her CA125 had risen.

The side effects after the third chemotherapy treatment were worse than after the previous treatments, but Jean handled it very well and she recovered quickly. *At times I feel guilty when I write or say "she did well" or "she handled it very well," because I was not the one feeling the pain and discomfort, I was not the one fighting for my life!*

After Jean recovered from the third treatment, we traveled once again to South Carolina, but this time she brought a new tool or skill with her—*Yoga.* Jean had taken yoga classes in the past, but she did not engage in it on a regular basis until a few months after her cancer diagnosis was confirmed. Even then, she was frequently so fatigued it was impossible for her to engage in yoga. By October 2005 her energy had recovered sufficiently for her to enjoy and benefit from yoga on a regular basis. Jean and I had been interested in meditation for several years and had frequently meditated while walking the beach, so it was natural for her to take an interest in yoga. But as it is with so many things, Jean and I approached yoga differently. I was interested only in the stretching and flexibility aspects of yoga while preferring to meditate without any of the physical aspects of yoga. Jean, on the other hand, wanted the entire package. Jean read about yoga, watched television programs about yoga, took yoga classes and she *"did yoga"* for the sheer pleasure it gave her.

By the time we traveled to South Carolina in October, she was doing yoga workouts on a regular basis and she even instructed a small group of woman on *"yoga positions."* She only taught yoga two or three times, but she loved doing it. Jean needed to find an activity that could be *"her thing,"* something she could be good at without any assistance from me—*and yoga was perfect for her.* Yoga does not require physical strength or much energy. It clears the mind, and it has a spiritual, even religious, nature about it. I have not heard of any physicians writing prescriptions for yoga classes or training, but I suspect that will happen one day. *Yoga helped Jean, and I am certain she will continue to enjoy its benefits for the rest of her life.*

We returned to Pennsylvania in late October, and Jean had her fourth treatment of the consolidation round on October 27. Her side effects were worse than they were after the previous treatment but still not as bad as she experienced during the first round of chemotherapy. *Oh God how I hoped and prayed this would continue.*

I prayed often for Jean, but not only for her. My father's health was declining, and he was continuing to lose mobility. I told Jean he would not last twelve more months. Also, my deceased grandson was still on my mind. I think my father's condition more than Jean's was triggering my memories of Lucas. *And so when I prayed—I prayed for Pop, Lucas, and Jean. I could do nothing else; every time I prayed, especially at that point in every Christian church service when you are asked to pray for those in need, I immediately thought of, visualized, and prayed for Pop, Lucas, and Jean.*

At the end of October we received the results of Jean's last blood test. Her CA125 had risen again and was now 9! Once more I was concerned about the increase in CA125. Was this an indication Jean's ovarian cancer had returned? I respected Dr. Goodman and his staff, so their previous explanations about the behavior of CA125 readings calmed my fears—but did not eliminate them.

I have many ways to determine how Jean is physically and emotionally. I measure her physical health by what she does and when she does it. When she says *"We are going out for lunch,"* she is weak but improving. When she tells me *"We are going out to dinner with friends,"* she is stronger but has not regained all of her strength; *and when she walks the beaches of South Carolina and beats me in a four mile walk, she has regained all her strength.* Measuring her emotional health is a bit more difficult, but there is one sure indication she is well emotionally. *When she gets up in the morning and begins to give me a long list of things to do, is critical of me for not doing enough and not working fast enough, … at that point I know feisty, five foot tall Jinka is back, and I should prepare myself for a few difficult days.*

By mid November Jean had recovered physically and emotionally and was once again ready to travel. And so for the fifth month in a row we took a trip to celebrate life. This time we did something very unusual—*at least unusual for us.* We planned a trip to North Carolina to visit my sister Elayne and her husband Jack:

Yes, North Carolina, not South Carolina! We did it at the last minute and we did not even tell Elayne and Jack we were coming! We spent the first night at a motel in southwestern Virginia. We could see there were still some *"fall colors"* on trees covering the distant mountains and we were hopeful about what we might see the next few days. The next day we traveled to our destination— Ashville, North Carolina. The mountains we saw along the way were spectacular. They were covered in fall colors slightly past their prime—but they were still breathtaking.

We checked into our hotel in the center of Ashville and were happy to have a two-room suite. As soon as we unpacked, we started our own walking tour of the area around the hotel. We found a beautiful old church that we loved and returned to on two more occasions. There were great shops—shops with character—and several interesting restaurants, especially a small restaurant frequented by people who lived in the area. After we returned to our room we called Elayne and Jack and make arrangements to visit them at their summer home. *However, there was one distraction: for the second time, Jean's hair was beginning to fall out. But Jean was so much stronger now than she was the last time this happened…. she barely mentioned the obvious loss of her hair!*

The next day we traveled at least twenty miles to Elayne and Jack's country home: a quaint cabin located at the base of a large mountain with a small stream flowing across the front of their one acre lot. *Their place was small but lovely, and Elayne prepared a wonderful meal for us; she is a great cook!* Earlier in the day they took us to two lookout sites on mountain tops nearly 6,000 feet above sea level. We do not have any mountains in Pennsylvania that come close to that elevation and the views were so beautiful I took more than fifty photographs. The next night Elayne and Jack spent some time with us at our hotel suite and later we went for dinner at a local restaurant.

It was a wonderful trip—spending time with Elayne and Jack in the mountains of North Carolina. My father would have enjoyed the trip, and he would have appreciated the beauty of the mountains. *My father and I loved nature, but mountains had a special meaning for us. Nature expresses itself in many ways, and for me mountains represent "power" and "freedom." But there is another reason I love mountains. Like many people, I feel God's presence in mountainous areas.*

When we left North Carolina, we headed east toward Myrtle Beach, South Carolina. We spent only a few days in South Carolina before returning to Pennsylvania for Jean's fifth chemotherapy treatment of the consolidation round. It was scheduled for the end of November. A few days later we were back in South Carolina. *It was probably December 3 when Jean called for the results of the most recent blood test. After increasing the two previous months, Jean's CA125 had dropped from 9 on October 25 to 8 on November 28. I was no longer concerned. Dr. Goodman and his staff were correct when they told me nearly two months earlier that CA125 readings do not signal a problem unless they exceed 20 and they are trending upward.*

December 2005 was so much better than December 2004—
the month we learned Jean had ovarian cancer. We spent two
weeks in South Carolina during which we did our Christmas
shopping. We had done this in previous years and always
enjoyed the experience. We returned to Pennsylvania in time for
our family's Christmas party on December 18. The party was
held at Suzy and John's house and we had a large gathering: Sally
and Dennis; Sally's daughters Tricia and Lori and their families;
our daughters Suzy and Lisa and their families plus; Jean and I
for a total of nineteen family members. *Claire (three-and-one-
half years), the grandchild of Sally and Dennis, and our grandchild
Helena (twenty-months) were the youngest members of the family
and they were both adorable.*

The next day was Noah's Christmas program at the Schuylkill
County Council for the Arts. The four year old preschoolers put
on a wonderful show. On Christmas Eve Suzy stayed with her
family and Lisa did the same with her family. We had a
Christmas Day gathering at our home with Lisa, Suzy, and their
families. We had a great meal with a wide variety of excellent
foods. We also exchanged presents and took many photographs.

As the end of the year approached, Jean and I prepared for her
last chemotherapy treatment. *On December 29 Jean received the
last treatment of the consolidation round. I hope and pray she
never again needs chemotherapy treatments!* The six treatments
of the consolidation round went smoothly, and Jean recovered
quickly after each one. There were some side effects to deal with,
but they were not nearly as extreme as those she experienced

after the third, fourth, and fifth treatments of the first round of chemotherapy.

What a year it had been. In slightly more than one year Jean had major surgery to remove ovarian cancer; twelve chemotherapy treatments; at least twenty five blood tests; she lost her hair twice (it grew back both times); a CAT scan, and physical therapy to help with some physical aspects of the side effects she experienced. It was a long, exhausting, expensive, and painful year that had ended much better than it began!

As the year ended we had two *"major issues"* on our agenda. The first was the CAT scan planned for January, which would give insight into the value of the consolidation round. The second was my father. For more than one year I spent far less time with him than I had in the past. I had tried to prepare family members, especially my daughters Lisa and Suzy, for my father's passing because it was clear there was not much time left in his wonderful life. I told family members that the remainder of my father's life would be measured in weeks and months, not years. I was always careful to add that only God knows in advance when someone is going to die.

CHAPTER 8

Possible Liver Cancer and Pop Dies
January 1 to March 13, 2006

In early January, Jean and I visited my father at the Laurels. He had been living there for over a year and a half. I told him it was too cold for him to go outside, so we would not be able to have a meal at a restaurant. He agreed, but he was disappointed; he always loved going out to eat. His mobility and his strength had declined drastically during the last six months and at times, he just seemed unhappy. He was also sleeping more; far more than he ever did. I remember visiting with him two days after Christmas when he ended our visit abruptly by saying *"I'm going to my room to sleep."* I had driven for forty-five minutes to be with him, and I was there about thirty minutes when he ended our visit. It was about 2 pm.

A few days later Jean and I again visited my father before traveling back to South Carolina. January in Pennsylvania can be very cold so we were happy to return to South Carolina where temperatures usually climbed to around sixty degrees during winter months. Shortly after we arrived in South Carolina, Jean called Dr. Goodman's office for the results of her last blood test. The results of the blood test, including the CA125 ovarian cancer marker, were all normal. We enjoyed ourselves in South Carolina once again. *Even in January, we loved South Carolina. I walked the beach—always barefoot—nearly every day, and I visited the fitness center at least five times a week. But now Jean came with me on many occasions. Jean attended yoga classes offered at the fitness center.*

It was a nice, relaxing, uneventful vacation, but we had several issues on our minds. I had a January 26 appointment in Allentown, Pennsylvania to deal with a growth on my thyroid, and Jean had a CAT scan appointment to see if her cancer had reoccurred. *In addition, we were deeply concerned about my father. We have a large extended family and many of them maintained close contact with my father. Family and friends called him on the telephone and he had visitors almost every day.*

Jean and I had maintained telephone contact with my father for years. We spoke with him by telephone several times a week, but if for some reason we forgot to call, we heard from Rosie reminding us of our obligation to call Pop. My father would always exaggerate any delay in our calling him. If I did not call him for four or five days, he would say *"Dear Lord, I haven't heard from you in months."*

One way I could tell that my father was slowing down was his failure to call me. He simply could not operate the telephone. In addition, it was extremely difficult to reach him by telephone. I didn't know if he was sleeping so soundly that he did not hear the telephone ring, or if he lacked the strength and hand—eye coordination to answer it.

On January 9th, 2006, some of my concerns were answered. My sister Rosie and her husband Pete went to visit my father at the Laurels and discovered he was seriously ill. They immediately rushed him to the Veterans Administration (VA) Hospital in Wilkes Barre, Pennsylvania. *My father was a veteran of World War II and was "removed from combat" during or after the "Battle of the Bulge."* During the battle, his feet were frozen, which resulted in circulation problems in both feet and the lower portions of both legs. These problems remained with him for the rest of his life. Because he was a WWII veteran who was injured in combat and was still experiencing results of the injury, he was entitled to a wide range of medical services provided by the VA. With the assistance of Rosie, my father utilized many of these services, especially during the last ten years of his life.

My father entered the Laurels in May 2004 and left there, never to return, in January 2006. When Rosie and Pete took my father to the VA hospital, his body was filling with fluid. He had congestive heart failure.

Rosie had *"power of attorney"* related to all of my father's assets and actions. This was reasonable since she was his primary caregiver. Rosie and I had many discussions about my father's condition and his future. I was certain that at some point the Laurels would not be able to properly care for my father. Where would he be cared for when the hard reality of his condition would force Rosie to remove him from the Laurels? The VA hospital in Wilkes Barre was always my first choice. Rosie, on the other hand, was conflicted about taking my father to the VA hospital. She agonized with the decision to take him there, but her options were limited. I rarely questioned decisions she made regarding my father. She frequently asked my opinion which I gave freely, but I always added, *"Do what you think is best and I will support you."*

Family members must frequently make difficult decisions regarding loved ones and do it in a maze of uncertainty. I am outspoken about many things, and I always reserve the right to express my opinion. But once a person, especially a family member, makes a good faith judgment, I will live quietly with the outcome. How can any reasonable person condemn someone who gave her best effort—*even if things turn out badly?*

Jean and I cut our trip to South Carolina short so we could spend time with my father. By the time we returned to Pennsylvania, my father had recovered significantly. And so he was moved from the VA hospital to the VA nursing home adjoining the hospital. I knew the VA hospital and nursing home were physically connected so that it was easy to walk from one to the other without going outside. In my opinion this was a major advantage to using the VA facilities. As I told family members, *"If Pop was in a nursing home during extremely cold weather, it would be very dangerous to move him in the event of a medical emergency. By placing him in an adjoining hospital-nursing home facility, that risk is eliminated."*

Now reassured that my father was in adequate, if not perfect surroundings, it was time to refocus on Jean's medical needs. On January 30, 2006, Jean went for her CAT scan. On February 1,

2006 she had an appointment with Dr. Goodman to receive and discuss the results and plan for her future medical care. _The CAT scan revealed a lesion (0.9cm in diameter) on her liver. Everything else, especially her colon and lymph nodes, were clear. After receiving nothing but good news for more than a year, it was surprising how well we took this major set back!_

We remained calm, asked many questions and I recorded notes. The most significant recommendations and information we received from Dr. Goodman were as follows:

1.   _The colon and lymph nodes were all right._

2.   _The lesion on the liver was 0.9 cm in diameter._

3.   _Ovarian cancer rarely spreads to the liver—It is possible, but not common._

4.   _Non-cancerous liver lesions are common._

5.   _In Dr. Goodman's opinion, there was a 30% chance the lesion was cancer._

6.   _There were four possible explanations for the CAT scan indicating a lesion on Jean's liver:_

     a. Testing error—it was possible the lesion did not exist

     b. Non-cancerous lesion

     c. The ovarian cancer had spread to the liver

     d. An entirely new cancer had occurred

7.   _Ultrasound imaging would not provide a better evaluation of the lesion._

8.   *A needle biopsy of the lesion was possible, but very risky. It would have been necessary for the needle to pass through the lung to reach the lesion, and this could cause significant damage to the lung. THIS WAS OUT OF THE QUESTION!*

9.   *A PET scan could provide better information about the lesion—perhaps determining if it was or was not cancer. I asked about the cost and Dr. Goodman said he did not know, but guessed it was around $5,000.*

10. *Dr. Goodman suggested we go to South Carolina and enjoy ourselves for a few weeks and after we returned, the PET scan could be performed. I strongly objected to that approach. I said "Do it immediately!"*

Dr. Goodman said it would take time to schedule the PET scan and it could take weeks for our insurance to decide whether or not to cover the cost of the PET scan. I said I did not care. I would gladly pay the $5,000. I wanted the test done as soon as possible. Later, I explained to his staff that I did very well with our financial investments in 2005 and into January 2006. I could easily cover the cost of the PET scan.

And then something happened which will probably never happen again. Jean agreed with me in opposition to the medical professional giving her advice! Reluctantly Dr. Goodman agreed and by the time we left his office, Jean had an appointment scheduled for a PET scan—for the following day!

We drove home, stopping first at our favorite restaurant for a nice meal. As soon as I entered our home I went downstairs to my office and called our medical insurance provider. I planned to inform them of the outcome of our discussions with Dr. Goodman, especially the PET scan scheduled for the next day. I also expected to argue or challenge someone about the need for a PET scan rather than the lower cost, more traditional CAT scan. I knew how to make the argument, including the merits of a PET scan. After a short time there was a real person on the other end of the line and I began. I gave my name and account number as required. The employee of our medical insurance found our file and was reading material while I began to make my presentation. I only spoke for a few seconds when she inter-rupted me and said *"Art, the PET scan is approved!"*

The next day, February 2, we traveled to Allentown for Jean's PET scan. Six days later Jean and I traveled to Allentown again for an appointment with Dr. Allen, a surgical oncologist recom-mended by Dr. Goodman, to address the lesion on Jean's liver. Dr. Goodman had told us Dr. Allen would be the best person to do surgery on Jean's liver, if surgery became necessary. And so we waited to hear from Dr. Allen, another very young, brilliant physician. He would give us the results of the PET scan and tell us what, if anything, should be done about the lesion on Jean's liver.

The PET scan confirmed the results of the CAT scan done less than two weeks earlier. This was devastating news because PET scans are far superior to CAT scans in one important aspect. PET scans more easily detect cancer in the human body by "sensing" the heat generated by rapidly growing cells. The PET scan results not only confirmed the presence of the liver lesion, it now seemed more likely that the lesion was cancer! Jean asked "How likely is it the lesion is cancer?" Dr. Allen said "70%." After giving us all this bad news, Dr. Allen suggested we travel to South Carolina and after we return, a follow up CAT scan or PET scan should be performed. This was exactly the same recommendation Dr. Goodman had given us only seven days earlier.

The next day we headed to South Carolina once again. The lesion on Jean's liver was a concern to us, but we had decided to *"enjoy life"* while doing our best to deal with her medical problems. More than a year after it was determined that Jean had ovarian cancer, we were both so strong emotionally and physically that even the possibility of cancer on Jean's liver did little to dampen our spirits or interfere with our lives. *I guess that saying is correct: "If it doesn't kill you, it only makes you stronger."*

Not only was Jean stronger, she now had a *"new passion"* a *"new thing"* that would come to entertain her and define her in the following months—jewelry making. Jean took a jewelry making class in January and another in February. Suddenly she went into full production buying tools and a wide range of supplies. She returned frequently to the store where she received the lessons and purchased supplies. There were always questions. How to tie knots? How long to make a necklace? Where to buy additional supplies? One day after a lesson, she returned to the store three times for additional supplies and more information about jewelry making. But what would she do with all the jewelry? She had the perfect answer: sell the jewelry and give the profits to the American Cancer Society. A little later she came up with a name for her line of jewelry: *"Courageous Chic Jewelry."*

As the end of February approached, we returned for a March 1 appointment with Dr. Goodman and we were loaded down with jewelry, a tool box filled with tools and supplies, and a strategy for selling jewelry.

We returned to Pennsylvania and learned that Rosie's ninety-seven year old mother-in-law was very weak, and like my father, she was coming to the end of a wonderful life. Rosie's husband Pete had been caring for his mother for several years along with other members of their large Italian-American family. Rosie and Pete had cared for their parents as they traveled parallel paths through life, and now it seemed appropriate that they were approaching the ends of their lives at the same time. Jean and I often talked about my father and Pete's mother. They had so much in common. But while we sympathized and prayed for both of them, we turned our attention back to the lesion on Jean's liver.

On Monday, February 27, I visited my father at the VA nursing home. I arrived a little after 1 pm and stayed for five hours. When I arrived he was very tired, but then he just *"perked up."* A companion Rosie had hired to sit with him said, *"He was looking forward to your visit all day"* and she added that he had a *"burst of energy"* because I had arrived. With each passing minute, he seemed to gain strength. But I could see he was experiencing pain. I saw half dollar size wounds on the backs of his feet, and there was a large open score on his lower back that I never saw, but I knew it was also causing him discomfort. He never complained, at least not to me. I was also concerned about his lack of mobility. During the entire visit, he never tried to stand or put weight on his feet. At one point two nursing home employees lifted him out of bed and took him to another room where he was given a bath. When they returned him to his bed, he did not even have sufficient strength to roll onto his side. The slightest physical activity was beyond his ability.

My sisters were expecting me to call them with my evaluation of Pop's health after I left the nursing home. But Elayne could not wait, so she called me during my visit with Pop. She was very talkative and I could not get her to hang up. Pop became agitated and said, "Tell her she is cutting into my time!" I told her what Pop said, but she just continued to talk. Finally Pop could not stand it any longer and he exploded: "Tell her I'm going to come down there and strangle her if she does not get off the line!" And so Elayne finally hung up, but Pop just made my day. His body was failing, but his mind and his personality were still whole. He was still himself!

Pop's evening meal arrived around 5 pm. He ate slowly, but he consumed nearly all the food on his tray. He also had two large glasses of juice. We talked while he ate and for a while it was like old times. Around 6 pm I told Pop I had to leave. When I was ready to leave, I held his hand and told him "I love you Pop." He looked at me and said, "I love you too." We loved each other, but that may be the only time in our lives that we actually said "I love you" to each other. It was such a wonderful visit, including Pop's reaction to Elayne's telephone call. There are times or events in your life that you never forget: some are good and others are filled with pain. I remember events of that day so clearly because it was the last time I saw my father alive.

On March 1, 2006, Jean had an appointment with Dr. Goodman. He scheduled a CAT scan for April 3, to track the lesion on her liver. He also scheduled a colonoscopy and an endoscopy. Blood samples were taken, but this time he instructed the laboratory doing the tests to check for colon cancer and liver cancer *"markers"* as well as the CA125 ovarian cancer marker. *As the appointment was coming to an end, Jean asked "What are the chances the lesion on my liver is cancer? Dr. Goodman thought for a short time and said, "There is about a 30% chance the lesion is cancer." We were happy to hear this because Dr. Allen thought there was a 70% chance the lesion was cancer.*

Two days later, on March 3, I traveled to Allentown for a fine needle biopsy of a growth on my thyroid. After the biopsy, we traveled to Sally's house where we spent the night. The next morning Jean, her sister Sally and I left for Myrtle Beach, South Carolina. We only traveled half way because Sally became ill. She had a stomach virus. The next day we completed the trip. Sally was sick for another day or two, but then Jean became ill with the same virus Sally had only two days earlier. Jean's illness did not last very long, so in a day or two the sisters were both healthy.

The morning of March 9, 2006 Jean answered the telephone. A good man's life, an exceptional life, had come to an end. My father crossed the river for the last time.

It took several hours to pack our things and then we made the eleven hour trip back to our home in Pottsville, Pennsylvania. We were exhausted when we arrived home. The next day we drove to the Wilkes Barre Airport to meet my sister Elayne after her flight from Florida. Marsicano family members were beginning to assemble to say their farewells to Pop. Later that evening Jean showed me a copy of the following prayer which she had read several years earlier and decided to save with the expectation she would one day read it at my father's funeral:

Do not stand at my grave and weep. I am not there, I do not sleep. I am a thousand winds that blow. I am the diamond glints on snow. I am the sunlight on the ripened grain. I am the gentle autumn's rain. When you awaken in the morning hush, I am the swift uplifting rush of quiet birds in circled flight. I am soft stars that shine at night. Do not stand at my grave and cry: I am not there. I did not die.

The Hopi Native Americans are often given credit for this remarkable prayer, which has been recited at funerals for seventy years. However, there is substantial evidence indicating it was written by Mary Elizabeth Clark Frye in 1932 and that she circulated it privately.

My father would have loved the prayer, and it does justice to the way I now feel about him and his wonderful life. I did not weep at my father's death, for even in times of sadness, my heart smiles when I think of him. *The above prayer also supports my feeling, or perhaps it is a belief, that Pop will always be with me.* My father had a wonderful life and he will be missed by the friends and family who loved and honored him. We will miss him, but even on the day of his burial we spent more time celebrating his life than we did grieving. This is as it should be, and we will continue celebrating his life, a life of joy, for as long as we live. Pop was a *"free spirit"* long before the phrase became part of the popular culture. He ignored rules and occasionally even violated laws, but only laws dealing with hunting and fishing! *This was something of a tradition in the Marsicano family, as reflected by one of my cousins making the following entry in the guest book at my father's wake: Pennsylvania Fish and Game Commission. My father would have seen the humor in this and he would have been very proud of it because he and my cousins loved hunting and fishing together—and they always did it their way.*

My father and I shared many of the same reservations about religion. In spite of this, I placed a copy of the following in his jacket pocket, as he rested in the coffin:

The Lord is my shepherd; I shall not want. He maketh me to lie down in green pastures: He leadeth me beside the still waters. He restoreth my soul: He leadeth me in the paths of righteousness for His name's sake. Yea, though I walk through the valley of the shadow of death, I will fear no evil: for Thou art with me; Thy rod and thy staff they comfort me. Thou preparest the table before me in the presence of mine enemies: Thou anointest my head with oil;

my cup runneth over. Surely goodness and mercy shall follow me all the days of my life; and I will dwell in the house of the Lord forever.

This is my favorite prayer and my favorite piece of literature in the entire English language. Even a person with little knowledge of religion will recognize it as the 23rd Psalm of the King James Bible. Shortly after I placed the prayer in my father's pocket, a Roman Catholic priest arrived and said a few prayers while standing in front of my father's coffin. We knew there would be a mass the next day as part of the formal Roman Catholic burial tradition. So when the priest finished, my wife asked if she could do one or two religious readings during the mass and the priest agreed. Then I asked if the 23rd Psalm could be read. Suddenly, I realized that the 23rd Psalm of the King James Bible is not the same as the 23rd Psalm in the Bible used by Roman Catholics. After a brief hesitation, the priest realized what I meant and made the necessary adjustment. I appreciated the gesture made by the priest, but the Roman Catholic version of this psalm is not nearly as beautiful or as moving as the King James Version.

The viewing was scheduled for March 12 and the burial for March 13. We had not buried my father when another tragic, but expected, event took place. Pete's mother, Mrs. Marko, joined my father on the other side of the river on March 12, 2006. My sister Rosie and her husband Pete lost two parents in three days! Jean and I had discussed the possibility they would face a double tragedy in a short time span because a very similar double tragedy had taken place in our lives approximately twenty-seven years earlier! Jean's father had died the day before our 13th wedding anniversary and my mother died the day after. Like Rosie and Pete, we lost two parents in three days.

The day of my father's funeral was very sad; the Marsicano family lost more than its oldest member; it also lost its "heart and soul." My father was a unique person in so many ways, but I always loved Jean's way of describing him "He is (now was) a real gentleman." After my father was buried, the Marsicano family gathered at a large reception hall where we enjoyed a meal, renewed relationships with family members and, above all else, celebrated my father's life, for his life was worth remembering and celebrating.

The day after my father's funeral, Jean and I attended Mrs. Marko's viewing. She was a remarkable woman I had known for nearly fifty years—since my sister Rosie and her son Pete married. She was a petite woman with an unshakable belief in God. She was remarkable in many ways, but it was her spiritual side that impressed me the most. I am happy she was able to maintain her personal connection with God to the very end by doing something she enjoyed, something which gave her strength: saying the rosary on her fingers.

As I near the end of my writing, I often think of Mrs. Marko who had complete faith in God and the Roman Catholic Church, and I compare her to my father who said he did not believe in God even when it was clear he had only a short time to live. They had this enormous spiritual difference and yet they had significant similarities. They both valued family above all else, they were the dominant force in their respective families, and they were both exceptional people whose lives had great meaning.

CHAPTER 9

The End of Two Difficult Years
March 14 to April 23, 2006

After two viewings in as many days, Jean and I headed to South Carolina once again. During our time in South Carolina, Jean bought supplies, made jewelry, and learned more about jewelry making. We only remained in South Carolina for eight or nine days because Jean wanted to take part in a fund raiser. There was another reason for us to return: Suzy was having minor surgery. After returning to Pennsylvania, Jean sold her jewelry, *her original designs*, at the fund raiser. She made a profit of three hundred dollars, which was given to the American Cancer Society.

Jean had a colonoscopy and an endoscopy on March 29 as part of the continuing effort to understand the nature of the lesion on her liver. Dr. Allen performed both procedures and afterward said there were no signs of any problems. *However, he complained that Jean had "solids in her bowel." Receiving a colonoscopy is not pleasant and I would imagine that doing one isn't either, so the presence of solid in the bowel ... Oh well.*

On April 3, 2006, Jean had a CAT scan to determine the status of the liver lesion. It was previously decided that a PET scan would not produce any additional or better quality information.

The next day Dr. Allen called with the results. The lesion had shrunk to 0.4 centimeters; previously it was 0.9 centimeters. This was good news, a smaller lesion must be better than a larger one. But the central question remained. Was the lesion cancer?

On April 10, 2006 Jean had an appointment with Dr. Goodman; perhaps he could give us a more definitive answer about the nature of the now smaller lesion on her liver. After Jean was given a physical examination, I was called back to sit in on the consultation. This was a very important meeting, so I took notes, as I often did. The following items were discussed in the order presented below:

1. *Dr. Goodman said he thought it was less than 30% likely the lesion on Jean's liver was cancer. He added that its pattern did not match ovarian cancer.*

2. *He said if it was liver cancer, it was Stage I; if it was ovarian cancer, it was still Stage III. (Dr. Allen had told us that it would be Stage IV ovarian cancer if it had spread from the original ovarian cancer.)*

3. *He told us the lesion became smaller, decreasing in size from 0.9cm in diameter to 0.4cm in diameter.*

4. *I asked if eighteen months was still the time frame in which ovarian cancer was most likely to reoccur. He said yes, it was most likely to reoccur in eighteen months from the time of surgery. (At this point it was approximately sixteen months after the surgery.)*

5. Dr. Goodman suggested the next appointment take place in six weeks.

6. Dr. Goodman discussed recent blood test results and reminded us that the last CA125 value was normal. In addition, the tests for other cancer markers related to liver and colon cancer did not indicate any reason for concern. I suggested that the next blood test include markers for liver and colon cancer, in addition to the CA125 marker for ovarian cancer. He recommended against including liver and colon cancer markers because there are so many false positives. However, he said he would include the additional markers if that was what Jean wanted. Jean said "no," she did not want the additional cancer markers included in the tests…. She was irritated with me for making the suggestion.

7. Dr. Goodman indicated that the next CAT scan would be done in approximately three months. He also said, "If the lesion grows significantly, biopsy or surgical removal would be considered."

After we left Dr. Goodman's office we did what we had been doing for fifteen months: we stopped at our favorite restaurant for a meal, called family and some friends, and reviewed and evaluated what took place during the appointment with Dr. Goodman. We both believed that things were good and likely to get better. *There was no certainty because certainty is not possible when dealing with ovarian cancer. Nevertheless, it seemed that Jean was winning her private war against cancer.*

We were still concerned about the lesion on her liver, but we took comfort in knowing the lesion shrunk. We also had a plan of action if the lesion ever began to grow or if it was concluded that the lesion was cancer. We did our best; we had outstanding medical professionals helping us; and we were strong. We were strong physically and emotionally.

Very little of any importance happened in what remained of the two years I promised to describe in this book. We went to South Carolina; we walked the beaches; Jean joined me at the fitness center on several occasions; we had dinner with friends; we went to church—together and separately; we had fun; …. And once, only once, Jean cried and said to me, "I don't want chemo again."

Part Three

LOOKING TO THE FUTURE

The past two years have been very difficult for our entire family. Everyone experiences difficult, painful times, especially those fortunate enough to live a long life. When facing adversity, uncertainty, and sadness, many people will express and even internalize one or more of the following:

- *How can God allow this to happen?*
- *Why do bad things happen to good people?*
- *How can there be a God when there is such pain in my life?*
- *I am so unhappy. How can I go on with my life?*

There aren't any simple answers to questions such as these. Indeed there aren't answers, just responses that can never be complete. Words may give some level of comfort, but it takes courage, patience, and inner strength to deal with adversity.

Experience of the last two years has made me wiser but not smarter, more patient and more compassionate. Now more than ever I realize that family is more important than all material things and living and enjoying the present is better than cursing events of the past.

After two difficult years, Jean and I are still alive, still happy, still together, and still enjoying life. We love family more than ever, especially our wonderful grandchildren, and yes … we still love to walk the beaches of South Carolina.

CHAPTER 10
Our Families

I have three sisters and no brothers. Mary Jane, the youngest, and Elayne the oldest, have lived in Florida for over twenty years. Rozann and I have lived in Pennsylvania our entire lives. My mother Helen, died almost twenty-eight years ago, after a two year battle with lung cancer, and my father died on March 9 of this year.

Because she was the youngest, my father referred to Mary Jane as his baby. Mary Jane's last marriage was her third and by far the best. It did not last very long because Glen, her husband, died of cancer shortly after they married. Mary Jane has a unique personality and at fifty-nine she is still remarkably beautiful. Today her "significant other" is Terry, a good guy who fits in well with the Marsicano family. I expect they will marry in a year or so. I did not have the opportunity to attend any of her three previous weddings, so I hope to give her away and dance with the bride the next time she is married.

Elayne is sixty-nine, and since my father's passing, she is the oldest member of the Marsicano family. After my father's funeral she began telling family members *I am now the head of the family.* Of course that is irrelevant *Because Hell has not Frozen Over.* Elayne has one child, Debbie, who was the product of her first marriage. Debbie is fifty and has been married to her husband Jim for more than thirty years. They are semi-retired and spend every winter in Florida on the shores of Lake Okeechobee. This works well for them because Jim loves bass fishing, fast boats *(they have one)*, smoking cigars *(he shouldn't)*, and good looking women *(that's why he married Debbie)*.

Elayne's second marriage ended suddenly and tragically with the death of her husband, Bob. Her third marriage seems to work well because she and her husband Jack have been together for thirty-one years. They are retired and own several properties in Florida and a beautiful home in a mountainous region of North Carolina. I always enjoy their company and the next time we get together will probably be this June when they will return to Pennsylvania for the 100th birthday of Jack's mother.

Rozann is sixty-six and lives in Hazleton, Pennsylvania with her husband Pete—he is sixty-eight. She had twins forty-six years ago … Roxann and Peter. In 1966 she gave birth to a second set of twins. Sadly they died shortly after their birth. Like their parents, Roxann and Peter have lived most of their lives in Pennsylvania, not far from their parents and my father. It should be noted that Roxann has five children and Peter has four. I am grateful beyond words to my sister, her husband, their children, and their grandchildren for the way they helped my father during the last two years. They were always there for him, especially during the last few weeks of his life.

My niece Roxann deserves special praise because she visited her grandfather at least five times a week while he was in the VA nursing home and hospital. In spite of her nursing background, attending to my father's every need could not have been easy for her. *She had a special bond with my father and she feels his loss deeply.*

I met Jean's sister Sally when Jean and I started dating. Jean and I were sixteen and Sally was twelve. She was wild. Not sexually or violently wild, she was just plain crazy! She was also full of mischief—as her mother would say—and always getting in the way. At least she was always in the way when Jean and I wanted to be alone. One of my earliest memories of Sally is watching her and one of her friends sliding down the steps from the second floor to the first floor on a mattress. She and her friend were not embarrassed in the least as they continued this while I sat patiently waiting for Jean so we could start our date. When Jean finally appeared she was embarrassed at her sister's behavior, but she had obviously seen Sally in action before, so we quietly departed. Of course Jean's parents, Claire and John Lindeman, were not present.

I shrugged off Sally's bizarre behavior and we had a wonderful date. I am sure of that, because we had many more. I figured, *"what does it matter, Jean has only one sister who is nuts, while I have three sisters and they are all nuts!"* It may seem convenient of me to indicate all of our sisters are *"nuts"* and imply Jean and I are sane. Surprisingly, I am not the only one who believes this. One family member, who will remain nameless, told me I am the only one of my father's four children who is normal. Then he added, *"And you are at least fifty yards off center."* As far as Jean's sister Sally is concerned, I can only say read on.

Jean is approximately four years older than Sally, but they look alike. If I am alone with Sally in public, people Jean and I know will often approach us and assume Sally is my wife. Both of the *"Lindeman girls,"* as I frequently call them, are around five feet tall, have great smiles and wonderful personalities. However, I am frequently told Jean is prettier and looks younger than Sally. Of course I agree, adding *"I had first pick of the Lindeman Girls."* This has become part of an on going *"family story"* with no basis in fact, but it has resulted in many humorous encounters. I enjoy expanding on the *"first pick"* story by adding that Sally and Jean's father, Huntz *(his given name was John, but most friends and family members called him Huntz)* approached me one day and offered me a large sum of money to take one of his daughters *"off his hands."* Continuing, I add *"I wisely took the prettier one, who was also bustier."* This always produces a reaction, especially from Sally.

For many years, Sally has been a fanatic about three things: *her hair, her breasts and shopping.* I could write an entire chapter about Sally and her hair; and it would require several chapters to describe Sally's compulsion to shop. It should be noted that Sally's desire to shop is accompanied by her habit of returning most of what she purchases. Usually this happens the next day, but not always. I have been with Sally during a Christmas shopping trip when she stood in line to purchase a jogging suit. Within seconds of completing the purchase, she decided to return the jogging suit and walked to the area set up for returns where she patiently stood in line until she reached the return counter. She returned the jogging suit, completing the *"buy-return cycle"* she has become famous for. Actually this was not as stressful as some of her returns because this cycle only required thirty minutes rather than a day of *"reverse shopping," ... returning purchases from the day before.*

Since the time I met Jean, she and Sally have had a friendly rivalry about *"busts."* I guess it is a *"sister thing,"* but I cannot understand how two women could have a rivalry, lasting more than forty years, over bust size. *However, Jean and Sally always did make a "big deal out of the smallest of things."* Naturally Sally was the one who took the most extreme measures. I recall an exercise device she purchased that was guaranteed to enlarge a woman's breasts. That's one item she should have returned—*it never worked.*

Sally has been married to her husband Dennis for more than thirty years. It is the second marriage for both of them. Sally had two girls from her first marriage. Lori, the oldest daughter, has a love for the culinary arts. This will serve her well (*no pun intended*) in her current position: manager of an up scale restaurant in the Philadelphia area. Sally's younger daughter, Tricia is a paralegal. I told her she should become an attorney. She rejected that idea and is studying to become a nurse while maintaining her full time position with a law firm.

It is often said "you can pick your friends, but not your family." Jean and I have many friends, but our closest friends are all family members. It has been that way for a very long time and it will never change.

CHAPTER 11

Grandchildren

Grandchildren are part of the family, but they are so wonderful they deserve special attention. If you doubt this, ask grandparents or even ask parents who are eagerly waiting for their *"twenty something"* or *"thirty something"* children to get on with their lives and have the grandchildren they are desperately waiting for.

Grandchildren satisfy a special need that many grandparents— or those hoping to become grandparents—feel very deeply. In my case grandchildren filled two significant voids. I missed too much of the day-to-day joy that took place when our daughters Lisa and Suzy were children. My career, making enough money to satisfy basic family needs, and eleven years of night school consumed most of my time when our children were young. By the time I completed my education in 1975, Lisa was eight and Suzy was six. I had missed too many of the precious years when our daughters were young. *I thank God that I was there, and will be there in the future, to experience these wonderful years with our grandchildren: Daniel (age ten), Maria (age nine), Noah (age four) and Helena (age two).*

Our four grandchildren refer to me as *"Pop Pop"* and call Jean *"Me Me."* Helena is only two, but she is developing a sense of humor that reminds me of Jean and her sister Sally. For example, she recently started calling Jean *"CC"* rather than *"Me Me"*. This is a reference to the *"Courageous Chic"* jewelry that Jean makes. Of course this is a joke she developed with the help of her mother. It is wonderful to watch Helena *"in action"* as she calls Jean *"CC"* and then laughs because she knows this is a joke we will all appreciate. *Helena's latest trick is to dance and sing "You Sexy Thing" over and over again.* She knows that this produces focused attention from all adults and some children in the area. A round of applause is always given at the end of her performance.

Noah and his sister Helena are about as different as two children can be. Helena is a tease who is always talking, and she has great difficulty remaining in one spot for more than a minute. Noah is always happy and smiling, but he is usually quiet, almost reserved. He can spend hours quietly drawing, making works of art for family members, or watching one of many educational CD's his parents have purchased for him. Sure he watches TV, but he does it with great focus, clearly irritated when Helena intentionally disturbs him. Many kids are described by parents and grandparents as *"smart"* or *"intelligent,"* but Noah really is brilliant and frequently asks questions or provides answers that surprise adults.

Jean and I were in South Carolina this past February when we received a telephone call from Noah's parents. They were a bit embarrassed because Noah asked them where Istanbul was and they did not know. They called me and I told them Turkey. Several months earlier, Noah had asked me what the word

"*beast*" meant. I gave an explanation but realized it was a difficult word to define or understand. After I responded, Noah pro-
ceeded to ask if a chicken was beast and I said "*no*," but I knew he
was not satisfied. So Noah asked about a series of animals *(dog,
cat, snake, lion, whale, ...)* trying to better grasp the meaning of
the word *"beast."* I was never able to provide him with an acceptable definition.

Like many children, Noah is interested in numbers, especially
very big numbers. One day he asked me how many birds I see
while sitting on the beach in South Carolina. I could not give a
definite number, so I simply said *"very many."* This was a mistake because Noah wanted a specific number. So he began offering some very large numbers for my consideration. He said *"Are
there a billion?"* Then he suggested *"a zillion!"* I decided to end
this line of discussion by introducing a slightly different topic. I
asked if he knew what *"infinity"* meant. He said *"no"* but was
clearly interested. I told him it is the *"largest number, even bigger
than a zillion."* I went on to say *"it is so big only God can understand it."* He immediately absorbed this information, so he
responded appropriately when I asked him to define infinity for
his mother. Later I asked him to define infinity for Me Me. He
repeated the information I gave him and finished by saying, *"It is
so big only God can understand it ... and Santa can also understand it."* He had expanded on my description of infinity by including Santa. I am delighted that my four-year-old grandson was
adding his own "spin" on information he had received about God.

Maria is our nine-year-old granddaughter. In many ways she is like her cousin, Helena. She is talkative, full of life, and loves to tease her brother, Daniel. Although she is a wonderful young girl, she is the most stubborn of our grandchildren. I recall once scolding her for misbehaving while visiting us at our home in Pottsville. She placed her hands on her hips and said *"Pop Pop, I didn't come here to be yelled at. I came to have fun."* Jean and I agree that time with Maria or Daniel is always wonderful. But trying to watch both of them at the same time is difficult because they fight so frequently. There are many times I would love to take Daniel and Maria with me for a day of fun, but I simply cannot handle both of them at the same time. This means that I frequently take Daniel with me for a day of activities such as fishing and working in the yard, but Maria must remain behind unless another adult joins us. I feel guilty about this and try to make up for it by treating her special in other ways.

It is easy to make Maria happy; it requires nothing more than snacks, desserts or ice cream. She eats snacks of all kinds, and she never ate a candy she did not love. At meal time she will frequently insist she is not hungry and reject everything that is offered to her. Once the meal is finished, she suddenly regains her appetite and requests dessert. In spite of her small size, it is rare when she does not request two or more servings of dessert!

Maria is slim and of average size, yet she is an excellent athlete. She plays soccer, basketball, and baseball. She also takes gymnastics lessons. *Last year she had an amazing seven goals in a single soccer match, and she did it with little effort.* She is just beginning to play organized baseball, and she is already a natural hitter.

Jean and I love watching Daniel and Maria play sports. But Noah is just beginning to play soccer and T-ball, and Helena is only twenty-months-old, so she is too young for organized sports. Daniel and Maria are involved in a wide range of sports and most days, one of them or both of them can be found playing or practicing a sport. There are literally periods when this takes place seven days a week for several consecutive weeks

Daniel is the oldest, most mature, and by far the biggest of our grandchildren. Daniel excels at wrestling, which he does as a heavy weight. Of course he plays football because it is a sport his father played with great success. Pennsylvania is known far and wide for success in football, and Daniel hopes to one day play for PENN STATE. Who knows, this could very well happen. This past year Daniel played a key role on a team that won their football conference title. In addition, his wrestling team enjoyed similar success.

Our four grandchildren have one thing in common. They all love to spend time with Me Me and Pop Pop. It does not matter how many of them are with us. They all enjoy spending time in our bedroom sitting, jumping, or lounging on our king size bed while watching TV. Even when the side effects of chemotherapy were overwhelming, Jean loved having the grandchildren sit in bed with her while she rested. There was no need to warn them about their behavior. They knew instinctively that Me Me was not well, and they were there to give her joy. No matter how sick Jean was, when grandchildren arrived she immediately felt better, and so did I. Even after they left, the happiness continued; we would always discuss their visit several times that day and the next.

Family gatherings with all four grandchildren are special times that live in our memories for months and years afterwards. Reviewing the enormous quantity of photographs taken during these events refreshes our memories and results in hours of additional happiness. I especially enjoy placing the latest photographs into albums that are conspicuously displayed in the office area of our Pottsville, Pennsylvania home. The albums are arranged chronologically by year beginning in 1960, the year I graduated from high school. There are even pictures from my prom, Jean's prom, and our wedding. There are also two unique albums filled with old pictures of family members taken as far back as 1940.

Our daughters, their husbands, and even our grandchildren are all smiles and laughter as they see how we looked more than forty years ago. It makes the thousands of dollars and hundreds of hours spent on these photographic treasures seem like such a small price to pay for so much joy. All my favorite pictures have children in them. Lisa and Suzy were adorable little girls, and I was able to capture that in so many photographs that are available for all family members to see. There are also pictures of Jean, Sally, my three sisters and me when we were children.

The most recent and most popular photographs in our collection have our four grandchildren in a wide range of poses. But the "best of the best" is an enlarged photograph I carry with me in a special folder when I travel and is on constant display in our home in Pottsville. I love that picture of our four grandchildren, Me Me and Pop Pop. Looking at that happy picture never fails to make me laugh or smile, for it exemplifies everything I value in life. There is nothing more important than family, especially the children.

CHAPTER 12
Mind, Body, and Soul (MBS)

Many books, television talk shows and pop culture communications deal with Mind, Body, and Soul (MBS) connections. But MBS means different things to different people. This is to be expected because anything directly or indirectly related to God and religion produces a wide range of firmly held views. Nevertheless, caregivers and people with serious illness should become informed about MBS and develop concepts and practices which work for them. MBS connections exist and can have a powerful influence on the caregiver and the person who is receiving care. If understood and properly utilized, depression and sadness can be replaced with joy or at least with acceptance. If ignored, the MBS connections will still operate and will still be powerful, but will result in a downward spiral of unhappiness and pain.

Even children can begin to learn about MBS. When my grandson Daniel was about four years old, I began teaching him about MBS. I told him he should try to develop a Good Mind, a Good Body, and a Good Heart. Going to school, paying attention to teachers, and doing homework were the things he should do if he wanted to have a good mind. I explained that a good body resulted from eating good food, exercising and going to the doctor for treatment when he was ill. The concept of having or developing a Good Heart was my way of introducing him to moral and spiritual issues. I told him going to church, respecting his parents, and helping others would be the best way to produce a Good Heart. I always expanded on the concept of a Good Heart by telling Daniel that a man with a Good Heart protects children, older people, and women. Lastly, I told him many times that the most important woman in any man's life is his mother. Daniel is a good kid and his parents deserve most or all of the credit for his Good Mind, Good Body and most importantly, his Good Heart. *This is not just my opinion; other members of the family when hearing of one of Daniel's acts of kindness have said exactly these words: "He has a good heart."*

It may seem odd that I began a discussion of MBS connections by describing conversations with my grandson. However, my godfather exposed me to these concepts the year I entered first grade. I was five-years-old, and yet I remember it clearly. My Uncle Pete was my godfather and I loved him as much as my parents. When my mother did not take me to the *"Greek Church,"* Uncle Pete took me to Sunday morning mass at Mother of Grace Roman Catholic Church. Once while we were sitting, a woman arrived shortly after the mass started. All pews were filled so she stood off to the side of the church. Seeing this, Uncle Pete taught me a lesson I never forgot and which I have passed on to my grandsons. *"A man doesn't sit while a woman is standing." I immediately stood up and offered the woman my seat.*

Standing there, I was so proud; my godfather was teaching me how to be a man.

Uncle Pete was 6 feet 3 inches tall and weighed in at over 300 pounds. He worked his entire life at Marsicano's Bar and Grill on Alter Street in Hazleton, Pennsylvania. He, Uncle Joe, and Uncle Frank operated the bar and lived within a half block of their place of business. My parents, three sisters, and I lived on Vine Street, two blocks away. I walked those two blocks hundreds of times with my father, my mother and, as I grew older, by myself. Anytime I wanted candy, soda, or a slice of pizza, I simply took a walk to the bar to see my three uncles, especially Uncle Pete. There was never a time I was dismissed because they were too busy. They always had time for me. It wasn't that I was special; they always had time for family, and all children, family or not, received special attention.

Uncle Pete was very large, very loud and very, very happy. He was always smiling and talking. He was so popular; everyone seemed to know him. It might seem odd that he took his role of godfather seriously, but my parents had chosen my godparents wisely. Theresa, my father's sister, was my godmother and she was a wonderful woman who always showed me great kindness. The home she and her husband Neil lived in was a beautiful brick house, only three blocks from my parents' home. I often walked there just to see her. *(It is surprising how much freedom children had when I was a kid. It is sad that today children can not be given the same freedom I had in my youth!)* Aunt Theresa and Uncle Neil owned a bar and grill on the same street as Marsicano's bar and Grill, and it was only six blocks away. My father worked there for about five years with my Uncle Neil after he returned from the battlefields of World War II.

Uncle Pete was a wonderful godfather and a great teacher. His spoken lessons were in a quiet voice with very few words and always at exactly the right time. But his best lessons were those taught by his own example. I was a junior in high school when Uncle Pete developed a problem with his leg. I was a kid and expected that the world around me would remain constant, only I would change, go off to college and one day get married. Suddenly my view of the world changed when I was told Uncle Pete's leg would be removed. His diabetes had been out of control and a sore had formed on his foot resulting in an infection that spread quickly. *Amputation of his leg was the only way to save Uncle Pete's life.* A large quantity of blood was needed during the surgery and family members were asked to donate blood. I am not sure if this was a financial, insurance, or moral obligation, but I immediately volunteered to give blood.

I was upset and apprehensive the first time I went to see Uncle Pete after the surgery. But there he was. He was still happy and still smiling. He had been through a terrible ordeal and yet he was not the least bit sad or unhappy, and as always, he was kind to everyone. He hugged his wife, Aunt Anna, and told her everything would be all right. It was obvious to me that he was concerned for his wife and two children. The next time I saw him was at his home above Marsicano's Bar. *He joked that he tried to lose weight all his life and in just a few hours he lost 30 pounds.*

I visited Uncle Pete often, especially after his leg was amputated. I don't know how he managed it, but a short time after losing his leg he was back behind the bar serving drinks. He was still his old self; always happy and always kind. There was no sadness or unhappiness in him over the loss of his leg. Many summer evenings my father and I would play cards with Uncle Pete in the yard behind the bar. If only the three of us played, it was ten card gin rummy, but if we could find a fourth player it was a seven card game. Everyone played for himself and the wager for each game was always a quarter.

Winning was not about the money. It was the joy of watching the reaction of the winners and losers, especially when Uncle Pete was the loser. Uncle Pete was not a good loser and if he lost a close game, he would think nothing of tearing up a deck of cards while pretending to cry. I remember him telling my father he did not mind paying for my father's house, but *"Why must I pay for Artie's college tuition?"* Watching Uncle Pete after he lost was so much fun we all played to beat him. Of courses we always made sure there were at least five decks of cards available prior to the start of playing because if it was a good night, Uncle Pete might tear up three or four decks of cards.

During my junior year at PENN STATE, I received one of those horrible telephone calls you don't expect and never forget. My mother called to tell me that Uncle Pete had died. (He was only forty-three!) I was devastated by the news. She waited until after he was buried to tell me because she knew I would have come home for the funeral, even though it would have been very difficult for me to keep up with my studies. I never questioned my mother's decision because she was only trying to protect me.

After his leg was amputated, Uncle Pete continued to teach me by example. Previously he taught me to respect women; help those who needed it, such as the elderly and handicapped; to love family above all else; and to be happy. After his leg was removed I, recognized how truly remarkable he was. After the worst experience of his life, he refused to be unhappy or depressed, he refused to be rude or nasty to anyone, and he did not blame God or any person for his misfortune. Instead he remained happy, kind, and full of life. He remained the best father, husband and godfather he could possibly be. The world would be a far better place if there were more people in it like Uncle Pete.

A few years after Uncle Pete died, his wife remarried. I was happy to hear this and I know Uncle Pete would have been as well because he always wanted what was best for his wife and children. When I see his children we always talk about their parents, especially Uncle Pete. And we always laugh. It is impossible for me to talk about Uncle Pete or even think about him without feeling good. Uncle Pete had a good mind and a good soul and they remained with him at the center of his existence until the time his body failed him. He showed that a person experiencing physical difficulties could be happy and could produce joy in others. Even today, more than forty years after his death, Uncle Pete's spirit lives on in the hearts and minds of the many people who knew and loved him, and they speak of him so frequently and with such love that it is difficult to believe he is no longer with us in the physical world. *Uncle Pete is in my heart and soul, and he will be until I am no more.*

Uncle Pete taught me many things about family, mind, spirit, and happiness; but I forgot so much of this when faced with the tragedy of my grandson's death. Months after Lucas died I was depressed and my body was failing me. I had forgotten how to be happy in the face of adversity. I had abandoned the numerous positive aspects of the mind, body, spirit connections and allowed only the negative aspects to remain. I did not curse God for the death of Lucas, but I also did not allow the good that was around me, and the *Greater Presence* I see and feel in nature and family to comfort me. Turning inward as I did only caused my depression to deepen. Six months after Lucas passed away I realized the serious physical problems I was experiencing were the result of my depression and could be cured by using mind, body, spirit connections for positive results. Exercise was the key because I always found joy in physical exertion. I began to do moderate exercise such as yard work and walking and after a few weeks, I gradually added specific exercises for my back and ankle. We still owned our lake house in Northern Pennsylvania, so I made frequent trips there. Once there I was able to take pleasure in the wonders of nature and the many outdoor chores I enjoyed. In a matter of weeks my mind and soul were once again healthy. My body required months to repair, but I had learned my lesson.

The last two years were difficult physically and emotionally for Jean, and I focused on satisfying her every need. She came first, but I made time to satisfy my needs as well. At times family members were upset with me for exercising while Jean was recovering from the side effects of chemotherapy treatments. I explained to them I could not care for her if I was ill or weak. I also indicated I was with her for every chemotherapy treatment, every medical visit, and I took responsibility for her many prescriptions, all financial issues, all shopping, and most of the chores around the house. Jean always understood this and encouraged me to work out at the fitness center, travel to visit my father and when we were in South Carolina, to spend time at the beach. My father was especially irritated with me for spending time at the fitness center. He told me *"You are going to hurt yourself."* Another time he said *"You will become muscle bound."* He was also unhappy with the pace of Jean's cancer treatments.

I stayed very close to Jean from the time of the pre-chemotherapy blood test and pelvic examination until the side effects of the chemotherapy began to diminish. This could be as long as ten days during which my only connection with my father would be telephone conversations. Once he realized this, he often asked me *"When will she be cured?"* I would politely but firmly tell him the chemotherapy could go on for a year, *which is what happened,* and Jean would probably need medical tests and evaluations for many years, maybe even the rest of her life. After a few months he stopped asking when she would be cured, and he was delighted when Jean completed her last chemotherapy treatment.

Taking care of myself during the last two years produced many benefits. During that period I never developed a cold, flu, or stomach virus, in spite of frequent contacts with my grand-children even when they were ill. As a result, I could always be close to Jean without fear of infecting her with an illness while her resistance was low. It also meant that there was never a time that I could not take Jean for a medical appointment, shop for food she wanted, pick up her medicines at the drug store, or do the many things she could not do for herself. My continued commitment to working out at fitness centers also produced an unexpected benefit, especially when we were in South Carolina. Jean and I have been exercising together for more than twenty-five years. For years we were runners—actually we were jog-gers—and we completed several ten kilometer races. *We always finished in last place or very close to last place.* After our knees and ankles could no longer take the stress of running, we became walkers, something we still enjoy.

Even when Jean was recovering from major surgery or from chemotherapy, she was still interested in exercise. Whenever I return from the fitness center she always asked how my workout went. She would also ask about classes given at the fitness center that might be of benefit to her. She was especially interested in learning about yoga and Pilates. *My continued involvement in exercise kept Jean in contact with it and, if things worked out well, would provide motivation and easy access for her to return to exercising with her "Rock."*

Jean and I have very different ways of using mind, body, spirit, connections for positive results. I rely on a well defined exercise strategy for physical strength and well being and my own poorly defined concepts of God and all things spiritual for emotional strength. Jean focuses on well defined religious practices and embraces all the traditions and rituals of the Roman Catholic Church. She speaks of God and *"her saints"* with great conviction, and they respond by giving her enormous spiritual and emotional strength. In the physical world, Jean loves a good massage and yoga. Jean also exercises. Even during the darkest days of chemotherapy, she did all the exercise her body would allow. There were days when she could barely stand, and yet she would still walk with me…. *at a very slow pace.* I supported her by grasping her right shoulder in my right hand while holding her left arm with my left hand. Using this approach, she moved very slowly and usually walked less than a quarter mile. *Today when we walk the beach she always finishes our four mile walk ahead of me. When I mention this, she generally responds by saying, "Yes, but you are such a slow poke." I love it when she says that!*

Jean and I draw upon our pasts and our very different spiritual and religious beliefs to build MBS connections, without which we would not have survived the last two years. Caregivers and those who are very ill should do the same. They should build a core of emotional and spiritual strength based upon positive aspects of their past; upon their religious beliefs; and upon the Greater Presence which is within them. They should do this with joy, no matter how bad life may seem. Even those who are terminally ill deserve to have joy in their lives to the very end, and they should share that joy with those around them. My father was able to do this and my Uncle Pete also did it. When my time comes, I hope to follow their example.

Who is to Blame?

It is 3 pm on April 18 and I am looking forward to a day of writing while sitting on the beach. During times of illness, death of a loved one, or other difficulties, it may be tempting to place blame; it may even be necessary. But if blame is placed, do it sparingly, wisely, and reluctantly for the very act of placing blame can have costs which outweigh any possible benefits. It is appropriate to place blame if it halts an injustice in progress, if it restores property to rightful owners, or if it results in a criminal being brought to justice. But is it wise to blame the surgeon, even if a surgical error was made, even if the error results in the death of a loved one? Because medicine is more of an art than a science, even the most gifted physicians will make mistakes. And what is to be gained, the error has been made, it is in the past. If the error can be corrected, focus on that rather than placing blame for mistakes of the past.

Cancer is a difficult foe to defeat and the fight requires cooperation among medical professionals, insurance companies, friends, families, the patient, and many others. The American Cancer Society and the people, places and organizations of God will provide great support and comfort and will provide it freely and in great quantities. In the ongoing battle against cancer and other serious diseases, it is absolutely amazing how the victims quickly bond together and in most cases are transformed from victims to survivors and then into heroes. Rather than placing blame, many cancer survivors give freely of their precious time and energy to help others, especially other cancer survivors. Many do it while facing either an uncertain future or worse, a certainty which means they have little time left.

Even if they lose their fight with cancer, as so many individuals do, it is wise and so very appropriate and inspiring for them to see themselves as survivors and heroes right up to the time they leave us. All of us have a limited number of days to spend among the living, and it is best that these days be spent in happiness rather than in sorrow attempting to place blame for that which cannot be undone! Most cancer survivors come to know this, but it is best to know it sooner rather than later.

CHAPTER 13

What will the Future Bring for Jean and her Rock?

I love it when Jean calls me "her Rock!" Anyone enduring serious illness or emotional pain needs someone she can count on through the difficulties she is facing ... She needs a Rock she can lean on. I tried to be all I could be when caring for Jean and it was not easy, but I would not want it any other way. We made this journey together and no matter what the outcome, we will continue into the future together.

Jean's 61st birthday was one we will never forget. She was rushed to the hospital emergency room and admitted with pancreatitis. The next day we learned that an attack like the one she had could be fatal. A friend who is a physician identified someone we knew who died as a result of their second pancreatitis attack. Jean's 62nd birthday was between chemotherapy treatments three and four. There was reason to celebrate because the surgery and chemotherapy treatments were beginning to work. We thanked God for that, but Jean was experiencing a range of side effects from the chemotherapy treatments that made it impossible to celebrate her birthday with smiles, laughter, and the overwhelming joy of family celebrating life.

This year life was so much better than it was for her two previous birthdays. Her 12th and final chemotherapy treatment was in December 2005. After that the side effects gradually faded. They may never completely disappear, but at least Jean is once again happy and full of life. We still worry about the lesion on her liver and several days ago Jean broke down crying saying she never wants to undergo chemotherapy again. This year her birthday was wonderful. We were in South Carolina, depriving our family, especially our grandchildren, of the opportunity to have yet another happy family event. But any guilt I had quickly passed because it was Jean's birthday and she celebrated it her way.

I woke Jean at 6 am and gave her a bag of presents and two humorous birthday cards. She loved the multi-purpose massage unit, two beach wrist watches, and a gift certificate for a massage. After breakfast we went to the fitness center where Jean spent thirty minutes on an exercise bike as part of a *"spinning class."* Then she completed twenty minutes on an elliptic exerciser and another twenty minutes of exercise while holding three pound weights. *When we left, she said it was her best workout in more than a year.* That afternoon she went for a three hour day spa treatment consisting of massage, facial, and pedicure. She didn't realize this treat was waiting for her when she arrived for what was supposed to be a one hour massage. Her dear friend Brenda gave her the three hour package as a birthday present.

A little later we walked two miles on the beach. The weather was wonderful so we remained there for a while and two of our friends joined us. We didn't stay long because we had tickets for a performance at Carolina Opera, a theater located just a few miles south of our condo on Route 17. The show was excellent and Jean enjoyed every minute of it. We returned to our condo around 10:30 pm, but there was one last birthday surprise. While Jean was in our bedroom changing into her pajamas, I came in with a birthday cake singing the traditional happy birthday song. I had picked up the birthday cake while Jean was having her spa treatment and carefully hid it in a box which I placed in a closet. *Jean blew out the three candles on the cake (that's all I could find) and we enjoyed several pieces of cake while we discussed the wonderful day we had. A birthday with small surprises and the entire day together … It felt like we were kids again. This was our best day in two years. Joy had finally returned to our lives!*

The reader may wonder why this day is included in the chapter dealing with *"the future"* rather than as the last day of a difficult two year period. Just as a week starts on a Monday and ends on a Sunday, the two year period this book covers starts on Jean's 61st birthday (*April 24, 2004*) and ends the day prior to her 63rd birthday (*April 23, 2006*). This may seem too precise for many readers. *The engineer in me calls out for precision and certainty, but only when it is possible.*

Another reason for using Jean's 63rd birthday as the first day of our future is because I was confident it would be a *"good day,"* and we both hoped for a long future together filled with many *"good days."* In the last two years Jean and I frequently paused and counted our blessings. We especially did this during the dark days when it seemed possible, even likely, that Jean would be one more casualty in the long war against cancer. Counting our blessings always made us feel good, but it also put things into perspective. When we considered our blessings Jean would frequently say *"We can thank God for what we have."* I would politely disagree and respond, *"We worked for what we have."* Perhaps we were both right!

We look to the future with much to be happy about. We have four wonderful grandchildren who have good parents. Our finances are more than enough to support us for the remainder of our lives, and Jean's cancer is under control and perhaps even cured. And we have a nice house in Pottsville, Pennsylvania and a wonderful three bedroom condo in Myrtle Beach, South Carolina, ideally located so that we can hear and see the ocean while eating dinner, sitting in our favorite chairs or while lounging on the balcony. I am grateful for the wonderful life I've had in Pennsylvania, but like many other people from *"the North"* my future is in *"the South."* I love the people, climate, traditions, and history of South Carolina. And the beaches of South Carolina have a special place in my heart and soul, for Jean and I found peace there during times of sorrow and we always experienced joy there. *Dear God, I love South Carolina!*

Four years ago, when we decided to sell our lake house in Pennsylvania and purchase a place in South Carolina, both of our daughters had serious reservations. Lisa, our oldest daughter, told me *"you must be senile to consider such a move."* Jean was not as enthusiastic about the move as me, so I received the criticism. Today both of our daughters and their families enjoy

South Carolina and spend at least two weeks a year vacationing there with us. Of course I frequently say to them *"I told you so"* or I remind them their father usually knows best.

Our grandchildren love vacationing at Myrtle Beach with Me Me and Pop Pop. Because vacation time is drawing near, they are counting the days that remain until they once again frolic on the beach. I will never forget how Daniel, Maria, and Noah reacted the first time they experienced the beach and the ocean. Helena was here twice last year, but she was only one-year-old so it was difficult to gauge her reaction. A year makes a big difference when a child is as young as Helena. I am certain her reaction to the beach and ocean this year will be totally unrestrained. Helena will also begin to capture memories of the beach and ocean which will remain with her for a long time, perhaps forever. I know her brother Noah recalls events from the two previous summers. Because our four grandchildren and their parents have had such wonderful times vacationing in South Carolina, there is little doubt they will continue to do so in the future.

My sister-in-law Sally and her husband Dennis vacationed with Jean and me in Myrtle Beach, South Carolina at least four times prior to our purchase of a condo in 2002. And then there were two consecutive years when our trips were canceled at the last minute because Sally developed heart problems. Thank God she recovered and is back to her old bizarre ways. My sister Rosie and her husband Pete have visited us twice in Myrtle Beach. Unlike Sally who is in a constant *"shopping mode"* or *"hair frenzy,"* Pete and Rosie are very low maintenance. They are happy to merely walk the beach and hang out in the condo. Jean and I have had wonderful experiences with Sally, Dennis, Rosie, and Pete over the years and the good times with them will continue as long as there is a breath of life within us.

Family members and friends have visited many times while we were in South Carolina and it is remarkable how many of them spent time on the beach thinking, meditating, doing yoga or simply connecting with their spiritual core. Surprisingly, *the Meher Spiritual Center* is located along the section of beach where many of them have found peace. The Center is open to people of all religions and was founded by Meher Baba in the early 1940s as a retreat for the renewal of spiritual life. *Baba was an Indian of Persian parents and he attached no significance to religious affiliation or rites, but he did place importance on looking inward—"help yourself in knowing your real self"—as a basis for establishing a relationship with God. This simple but powerful message is best expressed in the following words:*

When mind soars in pursuit of the things conceived in space,
it pursues emptiness;
But when man dives deep within himself,
he experiences the fullness of existence.

Meher Baba 1964

The Center is a wonderful place and I recommend it highly to people of all religions, especially those who are hoping to calm emotional pain. Several members of my family and friends have visited there and all found joy in the experience. Even my father, a man who may not have believed in God, was warmly welcomed there, and he accepted and enjoyed the experience.

More than twenty years ago, my daughter Suzy asked me the following question that I believe was part of a homework assignment: "*What would you do if you knew you had only a few months to live?*" I gave her a fairly detailed response that included checking my will, organizing my finances, and planning my viewing, funeral, and memorial. Now I am older and closer to the time of my passing, so I would like to add the following items to my list:

- *I would enjoy every possible moment with friends and family, especially my grandchildren.*

- *I would spend as much time as possible walking the beaches of South Carolina while continuing my search for a Greater Presence.*

Part Four

PARTING WORDS

It is natural to be unhappy in the face of adversity. Personal illness and death or illness of a friend or family member, are experiences each of us must face. At such times the pain and stress may become so severe or last so long that significant negative consequences occur. Those who are seriously ill often become so depressed they cannot function. They forget medications and medical appointments, they do not eat properly, and they have accidents.

Caregivers frequently focus on helping others for so long and with such intensity; they risk becoming seriously ill or even dying before the person they were caring for. *All of us will face adversity one day. It is best to prepare for it prior to its arrival.*

CHAPTER 14

It Is OK to be Happy During Times of Pain

Death, divorce, financial problems, health concerns, and a wide range of other common occurrences produce emotional pain in all of us. Initially we experience stress, anxiety, or depression. If not attended to, these problems of the mind will become problems of the body. Lack of sleep, chest pains, and shortness of breath are a few of the initial physical problems that may surface. Later, far more serious problems may arise. If we fail to take care of our minds and bodies during periods of stress, the consequences can be serious. After my grandson Lucas died, all family members involved in caring for Suzy and mourning for Lucas experienced depression. I was certainly in a depressed state although my emotional pain could not compare to the pain experienced by the parents of Lucas: my daughter Suzy and her husband John.

My depression was accompanied with related physical problems. Approximately six months after Lucas passed away, I began to experience severe back pain. This was in addition to pain in my left knee and my right ankle, which my physician was treating with pain medication. The medications had serious side effects, especially stomach pain and nausea. I dealt with the nausea by eating more frequently and by drinking soda. I needed soda with me constantly because I could not function without it. I was teaching at the time, and I was unable to complete a lecture without drinking soda to control my nausea. In spite of the medications, I still experienced severe pain most of the time, so I needed to take additional steps. I began using knee and ankle supports, which helped slightly. To mask the pain I relied on cold packs on both my knee and ankle. Every morning I stopped at a local gas station and purchased one or two bags of ice along with a newspaper. I put the ice in an ice chest in the rear of my vehicle and during the day I would periodically fill my ice bags. If my ankle was extremely painful, I would remove my shoe and sock and place my right foot into the container of ice. The ice treatments did not cure my knee and ankle problems, but they provided me with some relief from the pain. After some experimentation, I found an over the counter medication that worked better than the prescribed medications I had been taking. I was unhappy with the physician I saw for my knee and ankle problems, so I found a new one.

I remember my wife telling me I should be careful with the ice treatments because I could *"get frostbite."* I do not know if it is possible to develop frost bit by placing your foot into ice, but on several occasions my foot was numb when I removed it from the container.

I disregarded my own physical and medical needs from January 13, 2000 *(the day we heard the devastating news from Suzy's doctor)* until at least six months after Lucas died. Initially this was done because I focused on Suzy's needs and later it was because of my depression. It may seem strange, but the pain I experienced did more to lift me out of depression than any doctor or medication. It was easy for me to figure out why I was experiencing severe back pain. Like many men, especially men over age fifty, I have a long history of back problems. However, for years I had completely eliminated my back pain by not lifting heavy objects and by doing a fifteen minute back exercise routine three or four times a week. My back pain was the result of not doing my exercises for approximately eight months! I began exercising, and in a few months my back pain was totally eliminated. I always found pleasure in physical activity, even moderate activity such as walking and my back strengthening routine. So the exercise helped me in another way. It eliminated my depression.

Knee and ankle problems have also been with me for a long time, but they were more difficult to deal with. My knee and ankle problems were also aggravated by the long period of relative inactivity. Today I regularly engage in exercise focusing on my weak points: right ankle, left knee, and lower back. I avoid heavy lifting, take over the counter medications for pain and, best of all, I have totally avoided surgery, especially the knee replacement surgery one physician recommended! I also learned a valuable lesson. I must pay attention to my own physical and mental well being, even as I focus on the needs of others. I was able to do this the past two difficult years while assuming the lead caretaker role with my wife and providing some assistance to my sister Rosie as she cared for my father until the time of his death.

It is very difficult to be happy while experiencing physical pain. Steps must be taken to eliminate it, or at least reduce it. At times it takes only a series of minor steps over a period of weeks or months to reduce physical pain. This was certainly my experience.

For many people it is emotional pain that makes it impossible to lead a normal life while facing adversity. This is unfortunate because happiness is all around us, and it is certainly less expensive than medical care for depression!

My father was remarkable in many ways, including his ability to find joy or happiness in virtually any situation. All he needed was family or friends. If large quantities of Italian food were available, a gathering of family or friends was always a major event in his life. I last saw my father ten days before he died. We spent five hours together while he remained in bed. He was clearly experiencing pain from the two large sores on his feet and the one on his back. I never saw the sore on his back, but the sores on his heels were open wounds at least two inches in diameter. In spite of all this, my father never complained and we had a wonderful visit which ended after he completed a large evening meal. During the meal he joked with me, and he told me of recent visits by my two daughters and their families. We talked about our many times together and I described a party Jean and I attended the day before. It was a 50th wedding anniversary party for Harry and Marie, my wife's aunt and uncle. Pop knew them well, and I was certain he would appreciate the retelling of a story I told at the party. The following story is absolutely true and this is how I told it at the party:

Harry and Pop joined me for a two day trip to our lake home in Northern Pennsylvania. It was cold when we arrived and the sky looked like a storm could strike at any moment. After we unloaded our clothing and supplies from the car, I started on my work. The house was nearly complete, but there was still some inside work to be done. Pop wanted to show Harry the natural beauty of the area, especially since it was the first time Harry traveled with us to the lake. In spite of my warnings about the weather, Harry and Pop decided to take a walk. I was working for at least an hour when I noticed it was starting to rain and they had not returned. My concern turned to panic when I realized the rain was freezing on everything it touched, and I had no idea where they were or what route they had taken. I was calling 911 when I looked out the rear window in the direction of the county road. A car pulled up to the top of the driveway and the driver wisely elected not to drive down the incline toward our house. Harry and Pop got out of the car, and immediately they both fell on the icy road. It took them several minutes to walk and slide their way approximately 300 feet from the road to the rear of our house. They entered through the nearest door, the side door leading into the kitchen. They were both wet and laughing hysterically, because they had safely completed their trek. While removing their wet clothing, they provided similar accounts of their adventure. Pop said they were walking around the lake but when they were halfway around, they changed their plans and began following the stream that flows from the lake. They went a short distance and Harry fell into the stream, which explains why he was "soaked to the skin." They continued walking. Suddenly the weather turned colder and it started to rain. Harry and Pop were not sure where they were, so they decided to continue until they saw something they recognized. They came to a road and followed it until they saw a house. They knocked on the door and asked for assistance. The owner of the house was kind enough to help them and drove them back to the lake house. At this point Harry interrupted me and shouted, "Everything you said was true, except for one thing: your father pushed me into the stream!"

I told the story at the anniversary party and everyone loved it because it demonstrated the true personalities of these two wonderful men. My father paid close attention as I repeated the story for him. When I was finished, Pop said, *"That's right, but you forgot the most important point. I gave the guy who drove us back to the house five dollars and Harry never paid me the two dollars and fifty cents he owes for his share!"* Suddenly I realized my father's mind was still as sharp as ever because I did forget that detail, a detail that was worth mentioning because it added so much to the story. I told Pop, *"The next time I see Harry, I will be sure to tell him about the money he owes you!"* There is one last twist to the story. To this day, Harry insists that Pop really did push him into the stream. I would not be surprised because Pop enjoyed a prank and pushing Harry into the stream … Pop would do that just to create a great story!

When my father and I were together, we could always create joy or happiness simply by talking. If our talk included a great story such as the one I just presented, our pleasure was increased. As mentioned several times in this book, my father and I loved to carry on conversations while eating together, especially if we were eating Italian food.

I miss the lifetime of wonderful conversations I had with my father. God I miss him, even as I continue to celebrate his life. However, I see so many of my father's wonderful qualities in my wife. Both had great personalities, were very popular, had great love for family, and could find joy and happiness anywhere—as long as family and friends were near them.

When it was determined that Jean had ovarian cancer, we were both devastated and remained in a highly anxious state for several months until we saw that surgery and chemotherapy were working. Even during this time, Jean and I could find joy simply by being with our grandchildren. When we were not with them, we could create happiness by talking about them or looking at photographs of them. Jean could also find comfort in meditation and prayer. We both find happiness in attending church services. I especially like Lutheran services, but occasionally I attend and enjoy Roman Catholic mass with my wife. There were times when we cried together, but in a short time we would count or blessings and think of our grandchildren. Even as I write these words, it is impossible for me to think of my father or our four surviving grandchildren without smiling.

No matter where we are, our grandchildren are always with us. We call them and they call us; we write them and send them presents; and they send us cards and drawings although not frequently enough. We carry their photographs with us, and not just the small ones that fit in a wallet. I always travel with page size pictures of family members, especially grandchildren. And when we arrive at our place in South Carolina, Jean always places pictures of our grandchildren on the refrigerator.

Even in times of adversity or sadness, it is possible to find joy. There is joy to be found in places of worship, with family and friends, with nature and in *"journeys of the mind"* to times and places that put you at peace or give you pleasure. During the last two years my wife and father faced great pain, and I was there to experience joy with both of them in spite of their pain.

CHAPTER 15

Death Comes to Us All;
It Is a Part of Life

I have always been intrigued by the language associated with death, for it demonstrates the eternal search for God and a deep concern about life after death. This is presented most clearly and with great beauty in the 23rd Psalm that was presented earlier. Every religion and every ethnic group has a unique set of writings, songs and rituals that deal with death. *Death is a part of life; it is the end of a journey that starts at birth.* Life is for the living and it is left to the living to determine how the deceased shall be laid to rest and how their ending will be described and recorded. There are many metaphors used to describe the time when people die and I present a few below:

- *Pass or pass over*
- *Climb the mountain for the last time*
- *Walk with God*
- *Leave this world*
- *Departed because God needed another angel*

I love all of the above, but my favorite is:

• *When I cross the river for the last time.*

Perhaps it is my love for nature, a love I shared with my father, which attracts me to this expression. I can easily imagine myself crossing a river, and looking for loved ones on the other side, especially my grandson Lucas.

At the time of death, it is right to mourn the passing of loved ones, but if they had a *"good life"* and a *"complete life,"* it is fitting, proper and of great healing value to celebrate their life soon after their death and forevermore. *Life is for the living and death is a natural part of life, so each of us should consider the end of our journey, for it is coming as surely as the sun will rise tomorrow.* Those who know their days are numbered should consider their life and their death, and they should try to enjoy the time they have left. One of my uncles and a friend knew months in advance that they were going to die. In both cases they had terminal cancer. I saw my uncle for the last time, two weeks before he died. We had a wonderful visit and of course we celebrated his life while having an Italian meal. My uncle had made a decision not to receive any treatment for the cancer that would eventually take his life. He said he would rather die from his illness than live with the physical pain that would accompany the treatment. I always admired my uncle because he was an artist with a special gift, and he had a spirit which allowed him to enjoy life fully to the very end.

My friend had an amazing sense of humor which he used until the end. We attended the memorial service in his honor and it was wonderful. There were many tears, for he was loved, but there was much laughter because there was much humor in his life. By far the best testimonial of the service was presented by his oldest daughter. She told us that her father said the following:

> *I hope I don't die on a weekend; I won't want to interfere with my daughter's social life.*

The above is not the exact wording, but the message is accurate.

I am not a psychologist or member of any clergy. Nevertheless, I offer these suggestions as a way to prepare for death:

- *Every day try to do no harm. Do no harm to people, especially children and family. Also, try not to harm the environment.*

- *Every day try to do some good. Most of us lack the courage, talent or resources to do "great things," so focus on doing little things. Help the elderly or the disabled when you see them in public. Give time, money or resources to charity, for there are many people in the world, especially children and single mothers, who endure "lives of desperation." I know there are children in my hometown (Pottsville, Pennsylvania) who never receive Christmas presents. I do what I can to help them, but I should do more!*

- *Think about your life. If you are happy with your life, if you have made the world a better place, then feel good and continue on the same path. If you are not happy with your life or with your accomplishments, then change directions. Change what you are doing. Become a better person, become a different person. If you know a change is needed and you fail to make the change, you will regret it deeply and painfully as you near the end of your life.*

- *Enjoy Life. You owe it to yourself, to your friends and family, and to the Greater Presence which gave you the gift of life. It will also make you a better person.*

Given the events of the last two years and my age, sixty-three, it is natural for me to consider my own mortality. I have little fear of dying, but I must acknowledge concern for what I would leave behind. I worry that if my departure came sooner rather than later, members of my family would suffer especially my grandchildren.

In the last few years, especially since Jean experienced serious health problems, I have done my best to exercise, lose weight, address my medical problems and maintain a sound mind. My frequent visits to fitness centers in Pennsylvania and South Carolina have helped maintain what is left of my sanity and have put me in contact with many wonderful people. When in South Carolina I spend time on the beach every day unless the weather is extreme. Time on the beach helps maintain my body, clears my mind, and helps me in my search for *a Greater Presence*.

During such times I frequently reflect on the value of my life and I remember loved ones who have passed on: especially my father and grandson Lucas. I also think of how and when my life will end and hope my life will have meant something.

A life well spent is a great asset as one approaches the end of her time, for it gives great comfort to know that a life had meaning and value. Even family and friends will find it easier to say farewell if the life produced pleasure rather than pain and joy rather than sorrow. That is why it was easier for me to watch my father's life end than to experience the death of my grandson. My father had a complete life, one of joy and happiness. In contrast, the short life of Lucas is far more difficult for me to accept because Lucas never had a chance to grow and evolve into the wonderful man he would have become. His short life meant something to so many, but it would have meant so much more if he had lived.

CHAPTER 16

Strength, Joy and Peace from Nature and from Others

During difficult times it is wise to reach out to family and old friends, for they know you best and they have been with you during times of pain and joy. They will supply you with love to ease your pain and with wisdom to deal with it wisely. But you will also need strength, and they will supply that through a mechanism I know exists but cannot explain. Even during times of great desperation, time with friends and family can do nothing but help you overcome the physical or emotional pain you are experiencing.

In the last two years Jean and I have experienced great emotional pain. In addition, Jean endured extreme physical pain resulting from her illness and the treatments used to control it. *God willing, the treatments have cured her.* If only I could have endured the pain for Jean, it would have been much easier for me. *It was during this time of pain that Jean gave me the greatest praise I have had in my entire life. She said, "You are my Rock."*

She didn't realize it, but that simple statement made it much easier for me to face the difficult months ahead. I was trying to help her and a few gentle words from her gave me strength and helped me live with the emotional pain I felt. *What Jean said meant a great deal to me, but it also clarified something I was experiencing but did not fully understand: It is possible for one person to give another person joy and comfort, but it is also possible to give and receive strength.*

My wife frequently tells me I am too friendly or too talkative because I say hello to nearly everyone I come in contact with. Frequently I have long conversations with a person who a moment earlier was a stranger to me. It is amazing how many of these casual conversations produce words of encouragement, words of wisdom, or even new friends. I am delighted that many strangers I met the last two years have become friends. I meet many wonderful, interesting people on the beaches of South Carolina and in the fitness centers I regularly visit in South Carolina and Pennsylvania. My interactions with these people give me great pleasure and reduce the tension I felt building up inside of me on so many occasions. *I feel guilty at times because they give me so much, and I return so little. They do not realize it, but I could not have survived the last two years without them.*

I workout at a fitness center at least five times a week and on average spend two hours per visit. I do a wide variety of exercises that are designed to maintain my body and clear my mind. While doing this I have conversations, discussions, and even friendly disagreements with many members and employees of the fitness centers. They are absolutely wonderful people—every one of them. However, the *"personalities"* and *"cultures"* of the fitness centers are very different.

In Pennsylvania the fitness center is often noisy and rowdy, and
I love it for it reminds me of my youth when I "hung out" at the
YMCA and the local playgrounds. Most days I see my friend who
hits the heavy bag with incredible power but always smiles and says
hello. I enjoy my frequent conversations with the retired coal miner.
We ride exercise bikes next to each other and talk of family. Tim
Holden, congressman from the 17th district, is frequently there,
always polite and always ready to answer the many questions he is
asked by members of the center. Tim is a good guy and I vote for
him every time he runs, even though he is a Democrat. Frequently
I see past students there, and it gives me a moment of joy when they
refer to me as "Doc," as they did when they were students at PENN
STATE. The most entertaining people at the Pennsylvania fitness
center are the 300 pound power lifters who emit noises from every
orifice of their bodies while trying to lift 700 pounds. While these
large men may intimidate some, I have seen their gentle side, as I
did when they befriended a beautiful young woman at the fitness
center who was depressed by the death of her brother. She has gone
off to college, but I hope she one day returns to the center, for I love
seeing her.

The culture of South Carolina is far different from what I was
exposed to all my life in Pennsylvania. In South Carolina the fitness
center is relatively quiet, and the people are always polite. There is
calmness about the place which exemplifies the differences between
the two fitness centers. I frequently talk with the retired Marine
who is "always faithful" to the Marines and to his country. He is
there three days a week and when I see him we joke, talk about the

country, and share stories about our families. I frequently see a tall, slim woman. We rarely talk, but I am amused by her inability to deal with her hair, for she is constantly "adjusting it" while she completes a rigorous exercise routine in a business like fashion. I admire the cleaning lady who goes about her business with a quiet dignity and will speak to me only if I speak first. She is very nice, but seems shy. I frequently speak with a woman who was born in Chile and has deep concerns about the future of her native country. She is always smiling, but she has far too much energy. I wish she would slow down. A retired NFL player visits the center frequently. He treats everyone with respect in spite of his celebrity status. Of course, he loves to talk about sports.

The beaches in South Carolina are fantastic! Unless the weather is extreme, I find a way to spend at least an hour on the beach every day. I enjoy walking barefooted, something I do even in winter months. Feeling like I am a kid again, I fly kites and ride my bicycle on the beach. I also love sitting while reading or writing as the sounds of the ocean wash over me. *Like many people, I am drawn to the ocean. The ocean creates a sense of calm within me and it helps me believe there is a Greater Presence.*

I enjoy my frequent visits to the fitness centers and to the beaches of South Carolina. But I receive far more than health benefits and enjoyment. I also gain emotional strength. It is difficult to predict the future, but I will continue "working out" at fitness centers and roaming the beaches of South Carolina as long as I have the physical ability to do so.

CHAPTER 17

Final Comments

If you have come this far, our journey together is near an end. Experiences of the last two years have changed me, and so I now view life, family, God and myself differently. Even the act of writing this book has affected me because for the first time I have clarified beliefs I hold but have rarely expressed. And finally, I offer the following suggestions, all of which are consistent with material contained in this book:

- *Do no harm, and every day do some good; for one day you will be judged on the basis of what you have accomplished in life.*

- *Search your soul and your mind to discover who you are and what you believe. As many wise people have said, "Know Thyself."*

- *Bring joy into your life; your body, mind and soul require it, and it will make you a better person.*

- *Embrace family and friends, but not for practical reasons or material benefits. Embrace them because they will help you find your proper place in the universe and the path you must follow to arrive there.*

- *Consider your death. It is better to consider the end of life while you and your loved ones are happy and well than to regret your life when your time is short, and you are about to cross the river for the last time.*

Our journey is now over and I hope we meet one day;
Perhaps in a fitness center, on a beach in South Carolina,
or on the other side of the river.

978-0-595-41318-8
0-595-41318-8